Making the Most of Fieldwork Education

Making the Most of Fieldwork Education

A PRACTICAL APPROACH

Auldeen Alsop
South-bank University, London, UK

and

Susan Ryan
University of East London, UK

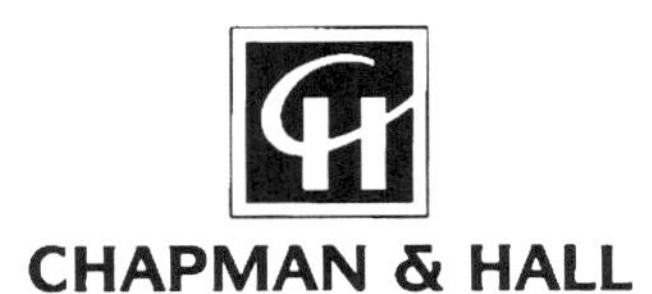

CHAPMAN & HALL
London · Weinheim · New York · Tokyo · Melbourne · Madras

Published by Chapman & Hall, 2–6 Boundary Row, London SE1 8HN, UK

Chapman & Hall, 2–6 Boundary Row, London SE1 8HN, UK

Chapman & Hall GmbH, Pappelallee 3, 69469 Weinheim, Germany

Chapman & Hall USA, 115 Fifth Avenue, New York NY 10003, USA

Chapman & Hall Japan, ITP-Japan, Kyowa Building, 3F, 2-2-1 Hirakawacho, Chiyoda-ku, Tokyo 102, Japan

Chapman & Hall Australia, 102 Dodds Street, South Melbourne, Victoria 3205, Australia

Chapman & Hall India, R. Seshadri, 32 Second Main Road, CIT East, Madras 600 035, India

Distributed in the USA and Canada by Singular Publishing Group Inc., 4284 41st Street, San Diego, California 92105

First edition 1996

Typeset in Times 10/12pt by Saxon Graphics Ltd, Derby
Printed in Great Britain by The Alden Press, Oxford

ISBN 0 412 60190 7   1 56593 439 3 (USA)

A catalogue record for this book is available from the British Library

Library of Congress Catalog Card Number: 96-84232

Printed on permanent acid-free text paper, manufactured in accordance with ANSI/NISO Z39. 48-1992 and ANSI/NISO Z39.48-1984 (Permanence of Paper).

Contents

Foreword

Fieldwork education, which combines work-based learning and assessment, has a pivotal place in professional education. It provides a precious opportunity to integrate the art, science and ethical practice of Occupational Therapy. The therapeutic milieu is also the most appropriate but difficult setting in which to judge 'competence to practise'. Yet fieldwork education has not received the attention, resources, research and status it deserves. This is why this book is so important.

The focus upon the students' experience reflects the central tenet of the book: the responsibility, challenge and pleasure of life-long learning. The book covers the whole spectrum of fieldwork in a way which will be of interest to academic and fieldwork educators too. This is achieved through a striking balance between reassuring, practical advice and scholarliness. The reader is encouraged to enter into current debates, engage in inter-disciplinary and international comparisons and appreciate the tensions between professional issues and organizational contexts. The insights into the logistical, political and educational factors which contribute to the theory–practice gap are noteworthy.

In my view, the authors have produced an excellent introduction to fieldwork education, and especially to the complexities of clinical reasoning which is a vital component of initial and continuing competence for many professions. I hope the book will enhance the effectiveness of fieldwork education and thus the quality of health and social care.

Irene Ilott, PhD, M.Ed Dip.COT SROT
First Alternate to the UK Delegate
to the World Federation of Occupational Therapists

Introduction: How to use this book

Our primary aim was to write a book about fieldwork for you, the student, to help you make the most of this essential component of your professional education. We also hope that fieldwork educators, academics and other professionals involved in fieldwork education will use the text to enhance their understanding of the experience of fieldwork. Our purpose is to provide you with information that will enable you to capitalize on opportunities that you have for learning during your fieldwork experience, and perhaps even afterwards, when you are qualified.

In these times of rapid change it is necessary for professionals to think, plan and act autonomously and take charge of their own affairs, but to do this they need a solid foundation of knowledge. We hope that this book will provide a means for you to develop that knowledge base and to learn how to use it effectively in practice. The contents do not, however, merely relate to enhancing your knowledge base. They focus on processes of learning to enable you to maximize opportunities and use learning experiences effectively wherever you are. We avoid being prescriptive so you will not find details of specific ways of working. Instead we try to help you to understand how the complex system of fieldwork education actually works and the role that you have to play within the system. We show you how to participate actively in the experience and so benefit from it.

First we explain how we have organized the book.

We have written the book so that you can read it straight through or dip into chapters that are relevant to your needs at a specific time. Each chapter contains what we believe to be essential information on the subject addressed. You will therefore find some overlap of material across certain chapters. At the beginning of each chapter we list the major points that will be covered, and at the end we summarize the main details. We have also organized the book so that it covers the complete spectrum of the fieldwork experience. This includes the preparatory time at university before the placement, the actual time while you are in the fieldwork setting and the period of adjustment after your placement, which might entail settling back into university or going forward as a qualified practitioner.

Sometimes it is hard to make a connection between all the components of fieldwork when it is new to you. Studies have illustrated how it helps to use visualization to gain an understanding of the elements of a situation and the connections between them. This is why we have used figures throughout the text to reinforce key points. You could draw figures for yourself, in your own way, as you try to understand the relationships between the different components. The introductory figure below illustrates our vision of the main elements of the book. We see it like a wheel with you and the fieldwork experience as the hub surrounded by all sorts of knowledge, organizational contexts and learning opportunities which are relevant to you in the fieldwork situation.

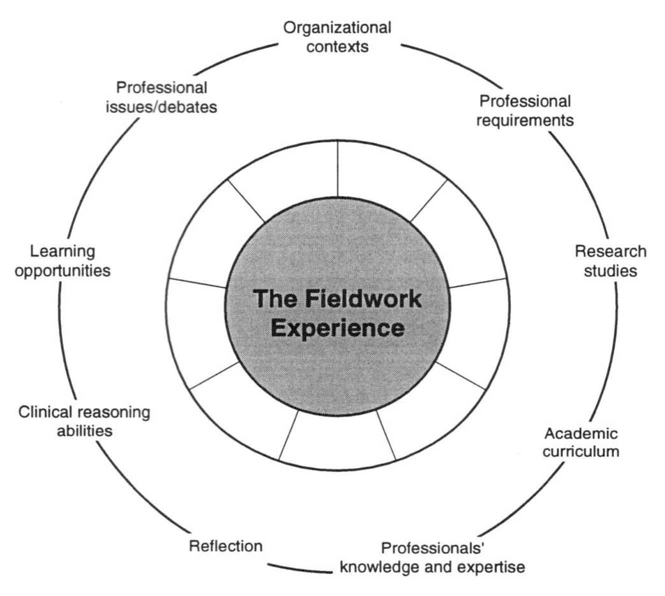

Introductory figure The wheel of fieldwork experience

The text is divided into two parts. The first part outlines the professional and organizational contexts of fieldwork education and the second presents the fieldwork experience in chronological order. We draw on material from a wide range of sources: personal experience, professional resources, published work, findings from research studies, literature about adult learning theories and professional development, clinical reasoning and reflection principles. Your needs and responsibilities and the process of professional development are examined in depth. There are ideas and exercises to help you enhance your learning and case stories help illustrate the points we make. Each part is now explained in a little more detail.

PART ONE

In Part One we set the scene and give you background information about fieldwork education. You will find this a useful reference at different times during your professional education. Fieldwork is examined from many perspectives. We explain how it is organized, how it fits into the overall curriculum and we consider the aims and purpose of this part of your educational programme. We then explain some of the current debates for the profession about fieldwork education. We try to present different perspectives on the issues so that you can form an opinion of your own. The chapters in this part show that fieldwork is actually quite complex, but it is an extremely important part of your professional education.

PART TWO

The chapters in this part follow the chronological order of the actual fieldwork experience from beginning to end. Woven into the text at appropriate times are chapters on ways of enhancing your learning, of improving your clinical reasoning skills, and of using reflection to augment the whole event. We highlight the things that you can actively do for yourself to maximize your learning opportunities and to ensure that you feel in control of the experience. You will also find that you can go back to the book at different stages of your education and use it as your needs change. You will find that you will need different kinds of information each time you go on a placement. Fieldwork education will make many demands on you. This book should provide you with the knowledge that will enable you, not only to gain the most from your experience, but also to give you the confidence to enjoy it.

In the book we refer to Occupational Therapy since we have written the book primarily for this profession. Many of the ideas are, however, transferable to other professions and could be used to enable students of other professional groups to gain the most from their own experience of learning through practice.

PART ONE
Professional and Organizational Contexts of Fieldwork

What is fieldwork education? 1

This chapter covers:

- definitions of fieldwork education, supervision and professional education;
- world and national professional requirements;
- the purpose of fieldwork education.

Fieldwork education accounts for approximately one-third of the total educational programme which leads to your Occupational Therapy qualification and to State Registration. It is therefore a very important component of your course. Your fieldwork placement is where you put your academic knowledge into practice and develop your reasoning and reflection skills, your interactional skills and your practical expertise. You can see this from the College of Occupational Therapists' (1993) definition which states that fieldwork education is:

> an integral component of the total curriculum through which the student is enabled to develop, demonstrate and achieve competence to practise as an occupational therapist. Fieldwork education complements, supports and informs academic studies and is undertaken as a partnership between a student, an identified fieldwork educator, and the education centre (p. 2).

The College of Occupational Therapists' Standards document SPP 165 (1993) explains that fieldwork education is a **process** which involves a partnership between the fieldwork educator and the student in the fieldwork setting. It offers an opportunity for rehearsal of, and reflection on, practice. This emphasis on fieldwork education as a process is the underpinning feature of this book.

In a moment we examine the purpose and aims of fieldwork education and suggest why it forms an essential part of the educational programme. In essence, the purpose and requirements of fieldwork education provide the agenda for the fieldwork curriculum within the course and, as such, provide the agenda for the book. First, however, we take a brief look at terminology and the requirements of the professional organizations which have an interest in the fieldwork curriculum so that you can understand the educational and professional contexts of the fieldwork experience.

TERMINOLOGY

In the literature the words **fieldwork education, clinical education, professional fieldwork experience,** and **clinical practice** are all terms used to describe that special part of the professional educational programme in which students gain **hands on** experience of working with clients under the supervision of a qualified practitioner.

Fieldwork is the term preferred by the College of Occupational Therapists and Occupational Therapy Associations in other countries. This is because occupational therapists now work in many environments and not just in clinics or hospitals. Education rather than **practice,** and **educator** rather than **supervisor** are the terms preferred by universities as these reinforce the educational nature of the experience. Hence **fieldwork education** and the **fieldwork educator** are the terms adopted and used in this book. Other professions continue to use the term **clinical** to describe the professional experience gained by their students. The terms may be used interchangeably although the subtle characteristics in these different terms should not be lost.

Definitions

These are the definitions that we choose to use.

Supervision:	The action process or occupation of supervising; a critical watching and directing as of activities or a course of action
Education:	The act or process of educating, coaching, tutoring, guiding

(*Websters Ninth New Collegiate Dictionary*, 1987)

PROFESSIONAL BODIES – NATIONAL

In the United Kingdom (UK) there are two organizations which have an interest in fieldwork. These are the College of Occupational Therapists (COT), which is the national professional body, and the Council for Professions Supplementary to Medicine (CPSM), which is the authority responsible for State Registration. In other countries systems might vary, but there is still likely to be a national professional association and an authority which deals with licensing or other legal requirements for the employment of therapists.

The College of Occupational Therapists guides and monitors the educational activities of the profession. For qualifying educational programmes, it takes its lead from the World Federation of Occupational Therapists (WFOT), the international body which sets the minimum requirements for Occupational Therapy education. These are explained shortly.

In the UK, the Occupational Therapists' Board of the Council for Professions Supplementary to Medicine is the body empowered through the Professions

Supplementary to Medicine Act (1960) to register occupational therapists and other health professionals. Registration constitutes the **licence to practise**. Registration assures employers and clients of a satisfactory standard of practice and acts as a safeguard against unnecessary risk. All health professionals identified in the 1960 Act, including those who have been educated abroad, must register with the CPSM before taking employment in the UK. Other countries such as Australia, Canada and the United States of America require therapists to take a registration examination before they can practise in that country.

In order to maintain quality and professional standards the Occupational Therapists' Board of the CPSM is involved jointly with the College of Occupational Therapists in the validation (formal approval) of all educational programmes in the UK which lead to State Registration. They take steps to safeguard professional standards by only recommending for approval those educational programmes which meet strict quality controls and legal requirements.

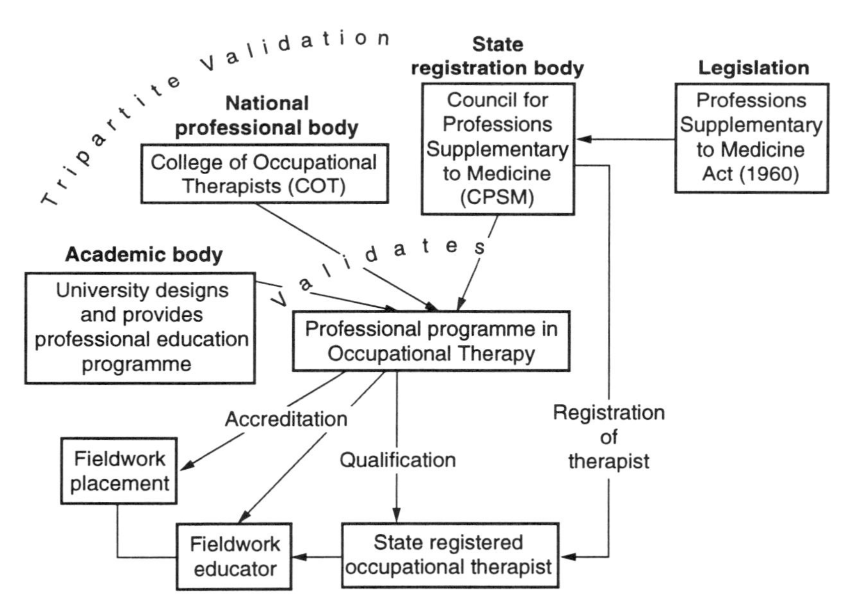

Figure 1.1 The relationship between the professional bodies, the university and the placement

PROFESSIONAL BODIES – INTERNATIONAL

The World Federation of Occupational Therapists is the official organization for the promotion of Occupational Therapy worldwide. Established in 1952, its functions are:

- to promote global cooperation within the profession;
- to promote internationally recognized standards for the education of occupational therapists;

- to develop and maintain communication with international organizations;
- to encourage regional activity between occupational therapists;
- to monitor constitutions of countries seeking membership of WFOT;
- to maintain and monitor ethical practices and review standards within the profession;
- to facilitate the exchange of information. (Occupational Therapists' Reference Book, 1992).

These WFOT standards provide an internationally recognized measure of the quality of training for occupational therapists. The WFOT standards for fieldwork require that:

- each student has a minimum of 1000 hours fieldwork;
- experience is supervised by an occupational therapist;
- fieldwork education takes place in a number of settings which provide services to individuals with different types of need;
- at least 50% of fieldwork education is completed on a full-time basis;
- students gain experience with clients of different age groups and with acute, long-term and degenerative conditions and in different organizational settings;
- each student receives a graded exposure to treatment through observation and directed practice, progressing to supervised independent practice with a caseload of clients.

The settings in which fieldwork education must be completed are not specified here. This allows some flexibility for delivering fieldwork education to reflect local needs and circumstances. It is clear, however, that recognition of, and respect for, the World Federation standards are crucial to maintaining the quality of education and practice of occupational therapists throughout the world.

PURPOSE OF FIELDWORK

In considering the purpose and aims of fieldwork education we acknowledge not only the aims specified by the Professional Body but also those which have been identified through research and practice and reported in professional literature.
The College of Occupational Therapists (1993) states that the aims are:

- to promote professional competence, confidence and identity;
- to provide opportunities for students to work with patients and clients and implement the Occupational Therapy process;
- to provide opportunities for students to integrate theoretical and practical learning;
- to facilitate consolidation of students' previous learning;
- to offer students the opportunity to experience new theoretical and practical learning;
- to promote the development of students' reasoning and judgement;
- to promote reflection on, and analysis of, experience and practice;
- to facilitate multi-professional collaboration.

Other writers suggest aims in addition to those above. For instance, Nystrom (1986) believes that fieldwork education provides the forum for practising problem-solving skills on which so much of an occupational therapists' work depends. A number of authors (Boud *et al.*, 1985; Cohn, 1989; Schon, 1987) believe that it is important for practitioners to gain a personal understanding of how theoretical principles are integrated into, and explain practice. The fieldwork experience allows students to witness and question the application of practice (Crist, 1986; Stewart, 1979) as well as to focus on the more practical aspects of delivering client care. Taking a still wider view, fieldwork education is said to allow students to gain insight into the reality of work and the pressures of the work environment (Alsop, 1991; Argyris and Schon, 1974; Pottinger, 1988; Wilson, 1986). Given these views, you might now begin to see why we choose to focus on fieldwork education as a process which contributes to the development of competence.

ACADEMIC REQUIREMENTS

All Occupational Therapy programmes in the United Kingdom are now established in the university system. In this book we use the term **university** to refer to all institutions in which Occupational Therapy programmes are delivered. With very few exceptions, the professional award is a bachelor's degree. In the move to higher education, the challenge for the profession has been to demonstrate the educational value of the fieldwork experience, and establish it as equal to academic studies within the university system. To a large extent this has been achieved by integrating fieldwork education within the educational programme and not treating it as a supplementary feature.

In fieldwork settings practitioners assume the role of fieldwork educators. They have responsibility for the quality of fieldwork education and are expected to become educators who understand the principles of work-based, experiential and adult learning.

PRACTICE PERSPECTIVES

Having dealt with some of the professional and educational requirements we conclude this chapter by suggesting how your fieldwork education might help you to view practice from different perspectives to gain a comprehensive picture of service delivery. There are four perspectives that you should explore, these are (1) the service provider perspective, (2) the client perspective, (3) the professional perspective and (4) the practitioner perspective (Alsop, 1991). By taking any of these positions you will learn about practice from a different angle. Knowledge of all four perspectives should enable you to gain insight into the world of care delivery as a whole. The key components of these perspectives are illustrated in Table 1.1. You might use this framework as a guide for asking questions about any placement and any service.

Table 1.1 The four practice perspectives

The service provider	*The client*
Influence of social policies on service provision Relationship between institutional and community care Relationship between the organization and other local services and agencies Influence of market forces People who access the service Identification of clients' needs Prioritization and rationing of services Caseload allocation Caseload management Information technology to support service provision Discharge policies and procedures	Causes of disease, disability and dysfunction Precipitatory factors The way that clients present Clients' functional problems Clients' perspective on ill health, disability and dysfunction Effects of disability on clients' lifestyle Associated psychological distress Opportunities and resources available to the client within and beyond the service setting
The professional	*The practitioner*
Philosophies underpinning service provision Therapeutic milieu Theories, models and approaches used Occupational therapist's role in the team Stages in the occupational therapy process: • referral policies and procedures • data collection and analysis • accessing, compiling, interpreting information • principles and modes of assessment • intervention plans • evaluation of intervention • documentation of work • communication of results	Therapeutic media available Indications and contra-indications of using media with clients Use of interpersonal skills with clients Skills of observation in relation to care Strategies to assist the problem-solving process Skills of clinical reasoning Skills of reflecting on and evaluating practice Professional use of 'self' as an occupational therapist

PERSONAL DEVELOPMENT

The educational programme that you are following will enable you to gain an understanding of specific professional knowledge, the associated practice skills and the theoretical concepts which underpin Occupational Therapy. Fieldwork education will provide you with an opportunity to work closely with people and to experience what it is really like to plan and implement therapeutic programmes, to make informed decisions with clients and to manage client care.

Fieldwork education puts you in a context where you can develop attitudes and interpersonal skills essential for professional practice. By this we mean developing a sensitivity to, and an understanding of, the needs of individuals, the ability to relate and communicate with clients in a professional manner, the ability to suspend personal judgements and values and the ability to operate without discrimination. It also means developing a professional approach which enables and empowers the clients you work with to make informed decisions about their future. Finally fieldwork education exposes you to the culture of the Occupational Therapy profession. It enables you to become socialized into the profession and to identify with its unique approach and ways of doing things.

SUMMARY

This chapter has introduced the terminology and some key definitions related to fieldwork education. It has set out the professional and academic requirements at a national and international level and considered a number of perspectives on the purpose of fieldwork education. Emphasis has been placed on fieldwork education as a process which facilitates the development of professional competence.

REFERENCES

Alsop, A. (1991) *Five Schools Project: Clinical Practice Curriculum Development.* Unpublished Report. Dorset House School of Occupational Therapy, Oxford.

Argyris, C. and Schon, D. (1974) *Theory in Practice: Increasing Professional Effectiveness.* Jossey Bass, San Francisco.

Boud, D., Keogh, R. and Walker, D. (eds) (1985) *Reflection: Turning Experience into Learning*. Kogan Page, London.

Cohn, E. S. (1989) Fieldwork Education: shaping a foundation for clinical reasoning. *American Journal of Occupational Therapy*, **43**(4), 240–4.

College of Occupational Therapists (1993) *Guidelines for Assuring the Quality of the Fieldwork Education of Occupational Therapy Students.* Standards, Policies and Proceedings, SPP 165, College of Occupational Therapists, London.

Crist, P. H (1986) *Contemporary Issues in Clinical Education.* Slack, NJ.

Nystrom E (1986) The Differentiation between Academic and Fieldwork Education in *Target 2000 – Promoting Excellence in Education.* American Occupational Therapy Association, MD.

Occupational Therapists' Reference Book (1992) Parke Sutton Publishing Limited, Norwich. In association with the British Association of Occupational Therapists, London.

Pottinger, J. (1988) The Practice Placement Crisis, Accreditation and Joint Appointments. *Social Work Today*, **7**(2), 29–30.

Schon, D. (1987) *Educating the Reflective Practitioner.* Jossey Bass, London.

Stewart, A. (1979) *A Study of Occupational Therapy Teaching Resources in the United Kingdom.* Council for Professions Supplementary to Medicine, London.

Wilson, M. E. (1986) *Clinical Education – Educating the Clinical Student in the Practice of Occupational Therapy.* Dissertation for MSc Rehabilitation Studies, University of Southampton.

Webster's Ninth New Collegiate Dictionary (1987) Merriam-Webster Inc., Springfield, MA.

2 The fieldwork curriculum

This chapter covers:

- fieldwork as a component of the total educational programme;
- structure of fieldwork placements;
- practice settings.

The academic and fieldwork curricula combine to form a complete educational programme which is designed to ensure that you develop and attain competence to practise Occupational Therapy to a level acceptable for State Registration. The way in which the two curricula are integrated varies from university to university. In this chapter we explain very briefly the different structures that are in place in universities for the delivery of professional education and the fieldwork components. We then explore the range of practice settings which might provide fieldwork placements to give you some idea of the variety of experiences available to you for completing this part of your programme.

THE STRUCTURE OF UNIVERSITY PROGRAMMES

Modular programmes

Some professional programmes are designed on a modular basis and comprise a designated number of discrete study units, some of which are compulsory, others which are optional. Choice in the programme allows students to determine the pathway they wish to follow to achieve the professional award. Fieldwork may be programmed within modules or as complete modules, or may be supplementary to academic units of study. Placements occur at different times during the course.

Integrated programmes

Some professional programmes are designed as integrated or linear courses where all students follow the same route. Professional subjects are introduced in the first year but are revisited in succeeding years so that depth of knowledge and understanding develops incrementally. Again, fieldwork placements are interspersed throughout the course, each building on the one before. There are advantages and disadvantages to both course designs which we do not explore here.

STRUCTURE OF FIELDWORK PLACEMENTS

The fieldwork programme

As we mentioned in the previous chapter, the World Federation of Occupational Therapists (WFOT) requires students to complete a minimum 1000 hours fieldwork experience with a qualified therapist. Each university designs its own academic and fieldwork programme and so the length and number of placements which make up the 1000 hours vary from course to course. Some universities arrange the first fieldwork experience as a series of separate days spent over a number of weeks at one placement. This provides exposure to practice so that a student can start to socialize into the profession and make interpretations of practice. The hours may not count towards the required 1000 hours because the student is not actually practising. Most fieldwork placements, however, are undertaken on a full time basis and last anything from 3 to 12 weeks. These allow students to become active members of the team and to participate in service delivery. Students will have between three and five placements during their course to complete the required hours.

While universities in the UK programme a number of short- to medium-term placements, a model common in other countries such as the United States is that of an internship. Following an introductory placement, called a Level One placement, students undertake a long block of fieldwork, known as the Level Two fieldwork experience, at the end of their academic programme.

Practice settings

Occupational therapists work in a wide range of settings which is increasing as professional roles and fields of practice expand and change. Therapists are not only working as clinicians, educators, managers, and researchers, but also as consultants, advocates and advisors on social policy and on health and environmental issues. They work in a variety of settings for instance, statutory agencies, voluntary organizations, and private services. They also work in hospitals, health centres, nursing homes, day centres, schools, prisons, and voluntary and charitable agencies. Some therapists coordinate services across different settings, others act as case or care managers to coordinate services for individual clients. Therapists work with people with different problems such as mental health problems and learning difficulties as well as with individuals with physical and psychosocial problems. They also work with people from different age groups and with those who need different levels of care.

The focus of Occupational Therapy practice is changing so that it now includes primary, secondary as well as tertiary care. Primary care includes health education and programmes to avert or delay the onset of other problems such as social isolation. Secondary care includes treatment, education and interventions that restore and optimize function. Tertiary care involves maintaining altered function by, perhaps, adapting the environment for a client, improving clients' access to work, leisure or sports facilities, or adapting equipment that a client needs to use. Some services provide a limited range of services and refer people on to others according to need. Other services provide a continuum of care across different environments. Table 2.1 shows an example of paediatric services organized as a continuum of care.

Table 2.1 The paediatric continuum of service

	PREVENTION		HABILITATION *Interventions/treatments*		REHABILITATION *Training*	*Adaptations*
TYPE OF SERVICE	Screening babies for developmental lags Establishing bonding between mothers and babies	Sensory stimulation with neonates Feeding – premature babies Positioning and equipment for high risk neonates	Sensory – awareness Snoezelen Sensory stimulation Assessing ● babies who fail to thrive ● cerebral dysfunction ● cognitive functioning ● hand functions ● neuro-motor problems ● visual motor problems Acquisition of ● social skills ● play skills Group work with parents and children Working with parents as co-therapists Support groups for parents	Drama therapy Dysphagia ● oral motor problems Hand functioning Play therapy Perceptual motor disorders ● handwriting Psychiatric problems Sensory Integration therapy ● reflex integration ● balance reactions ● crossing midline ● form perceptions ● praxis problems ● visuo-spatial problems ● visual motor problems ● tactile defensiveness Sexual abuse counselling and therapy	Behaviour modification programmes Sexual habilitation/ training Self catheterization training Computer assisted programmes Community centre management Relaxation training Splinting ● static ● dynamic Serial casting Prosthesis	Environment ● playgrounds ● transport Integration/Inclusion ● in schools ● in community Adapted ● bathing aids ● classroom aids ● clothing ● communication devices ● eating equipment ● leisure/equipment ● seating ● switches ● toys ● writing equipment
VENUES	Hospitals Intensive care units Child health centres		Play schools Child development centres Homes Residential centres	Schools Clinics Child development centres Rehabilitation centres Hospices	Homes Residential centres Outpatients clinics	Community places Schools Homes

Sources: Paediatric articles published in *The American Journal of Occupational Therapy* and *The British Journal of Occupational Therapy*, 1982–94

You can, perhaps, begin to see the range of services in which occupational therapists work and which might provide fieldwork placements. Figure 2.1 illustrates the professional development opportunities available when you qualify. Practice is becoming more complex and it is evident that an undergraduate programme can only provide a limited range of experiences which serve as a foundation for practice, and on which you can subsequently build. Continuing education after qualification is therefore vital to your own development and to the advancement of the profession.

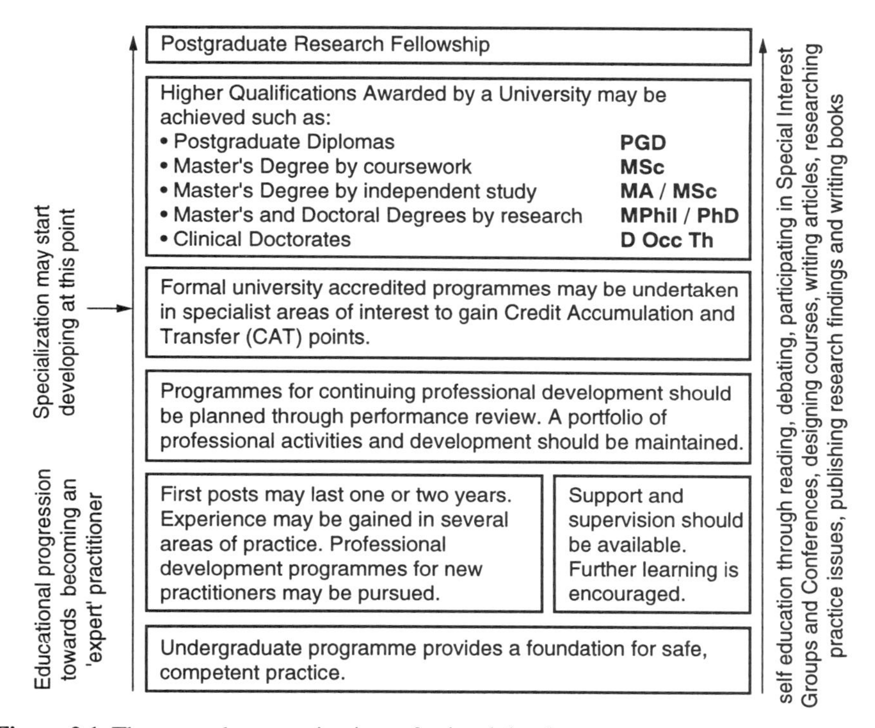

Figure 2.1 The upward progression in professional development

SUMMARY

This chapter has described the common structures used in the design of Occupational Therapy programmes and shown how fieldwork is provided within the total programme of professional education. The chapter has also indicated the variety of settings in which occupational therapists now work and illustrated the settings which might potentially provide fieldwork placements for students.

3 Fieldwork dynamics

This chapter covers:

- the changing nature of professional practice;
- how to gain a balance of professional experience;
- an overview of the principles and processes of practice

One of the most important things for you to realize is that practice is dynamic and offers both challenges and opportunities. Situations and demands are changing constantly, in fact, nothing stands still. Those who think that practice does or should stand still will find themselves falling behind! In many ways you need to get used to the idea of ambiguity in practice and to having to modify your views and adapt to changing circumstances as they arise. This is why your educators want you to appreciate the principles and processes of the profession so that you can work creatively in different settings and modify your practice to reflect new developments.

Schon (1987) believes that practice is like living on swampy ground, it is uncertain, unreliable, and messy. This can be worrying for those who are in it. It would be easy to ignore internal and external factors that impinge on practice and threaten to destabilize it, but realistically this is not possible. We are part of an evolving profession which has to change to suit changing needs and circumstances, however unsettling this may be. Figure 3.1 illustrates some of the internal and external factors which we must take into account in our work.

It is worth pointing out that change is happening in many health professions. Changes in health and social care systems can have a significant impact on the way in which any profession functions. Often therapists believe that change is peculiar to their own profession but this is not so.

THE SHIFTING EMPHASIS OF FIELDWORK EDUCATION

Fieldwork education has changed over time. It has moved away from focusing on students' practice and skill development to a system of education which facilitates students' personal growth and understanding of practice. It has moved away from a technical rational model, where the emphasis was on **doing** and on perfecting skills

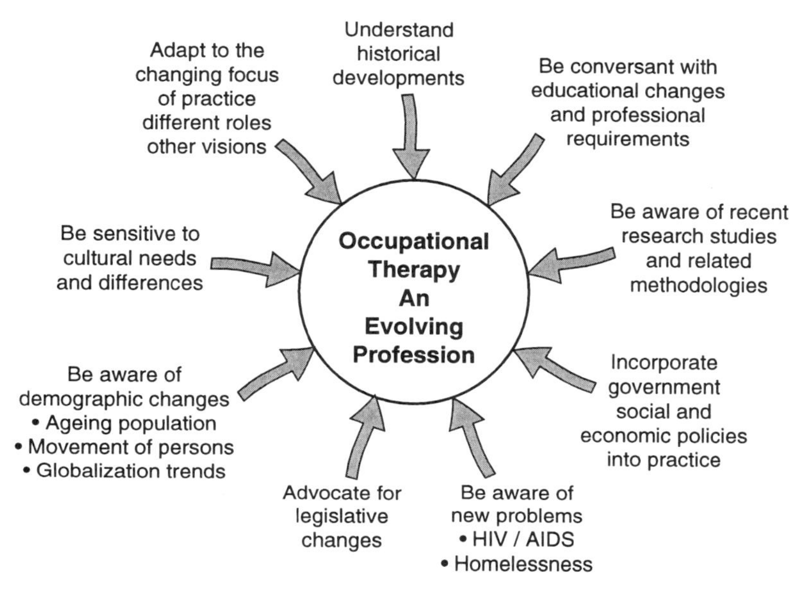

Figure 3.1 The changing profession: influencing factors

through observation, trial and error and rehearsal. Now there is a model of education which encourages **artistry** where the practitioner uses therapy creatively in different situations to meet individual need and circumstances. Fish *et al.* (1991) and Schon (1987) prefer to think of a practitioner as an artist who can alter and shift focus as the need arises. This concept may be quite difficult to grasp, especially if you have yet to come to terms with the fundamentals of practice. Table 3.1 shows the difference between professionalism as a **technical-rational** activity and professionalism as a **practical art**.

Reading through these lists may not make much sense to you at the moment but it is important for you to appreciate that there are two very different ways of operating in practice which can affect both the way you think and the way you work.

One way of looking at this is to think about people painting. One person may follow directions already laid down by someone else and fill in the spaces with the correct colours. This method of 'painting by numbers' prescribes the rules. Assuming the person's skills are good enough, he or she will produce an acceptable painting. Technically it will look good but the painter may not have had much to think about in its production. If required to repeat the operation, he or she could become bored and might feel somewhat controlled. Some therapists practise in this way. Their programmes and groups follow set patterns and theoretical frameworks as they strive for a satisfactory end result. This way of practising is fairly easy to manage but does not allow for individualization of either the client's programme or the therapist's work.

As you look at the second list, you might visualize a professional artist. This is someone who has learnt the rules of painting but operates beyond those rules to

Table 3.1 Two models of professionalism

The technical rational view	*The practical artistry view*
Follows rules, laws, schedules; uses routines, prescriptions	Starts where rules fade; sees patterns, frameworks
Uses diagnosis/analysis to think about teaching	Uses interpretation and appreciation to think about teaching
Wants efficient systems	Wants creativity and room to be wrong
Sees knowledge as graspable, permanent	Sees knowledge as temporary, dynamic, problematic
Theory is applied to practice	Theory emerges from practice
Visible performance is central	There is more to it than surface features
Setting out and testing for basic competences is vital	There is more to teaching than the sum of the parts
Technical expertise is all	Professional judgement counts
Sees professional activities as masterable	Sees mystery at the heart of professional activities
Emphasizes the known	Embraces uncertainty
Standards must be fixed; standards are measurable; standards must be controlled	That which is most easily fixed and measurable is also trivial – professionals should be trusted
Emphasizes assessment, appraisal, inspection, accreditation	Emphasizes investigation, reflection, deliberation
Change must be managed from outside	Professionals can develop from inside
Quality is really about quantity of that which is easily measurable	Quality comes from deepening insight into one's values, priorities, actions
Technical accountability	Professional answerability
This is training	This is education
Takes the instrumental view of learning	Sees education as intrinsically worthwhile

Reprinted with permission from the Editorial Director, David Fulton Publishers, London.
Source: reprinted from the text of Fish, D. (1995) *Quality Mentoring for Student Teachers: A Principled Approach to Practice.* David Fulton; London.

produce an individualized piece of work which shows high levels of skill and creative ability. Some people admire this ability, others profess not to understand. Some therapists work in this way. They adapt and use several different ways of working, depending on the client's needs. They feel quite comfortable about modifying their method of working to meet changing needs and circumstances, or as new knowledge emerges. They reach agreed therapeutic goals through a variety of means.

At an early stage in your fieldwork placement it might help to draw a framework or model to help you visualize and understand the processes you are using in that setting. Try to involve your fieldwork educator and draw the map together so that you both set out a clear representation of what practice in that setting is all about.

THE BALANCE OF EXPERIENCE

We have argued so far that practice is becoming more complicated, employment settings are becoming more diverse, and the roles of therapists are changing. It therefore follows that having only three or four fieldwork experiences before you qualify will not allow you to learn everything you need to know. You will only be provided with a flavour of practice. But what about standards and requirements for becoming competent to practise?

The profession has always recommended that a student gains a balance of experience between physical and mental health settings. But it is now considered more important for a student to develop the confidence to understand and use principles and processes underlying professional practice by gaining experience in various settings. Some knowledge and skills are transferable from one setting to another but many are not (Maxim and Dielman, 1987; Patel and Cranton, 1983; Tanner *et al.*, 1987). Table 3.2 shows which knowledge and skills these authors think are task specific to particular settings and which are generalizable across all types of settings.

Table 3.2 The specificity and generalizability of knowledge and skills

KNOWLEDGE ND SKILLS

Task specific to one setting	*Generalizable across settings*
Factual background knowledge	Attitude to health care
Assessments	Professional responsibility and behaviour
Problem-solving	Selection of data acquisition
Decision-making	History taking and interviews
Accuracy of judgement	Interpersonal skills
Evaluations	Technical skills

Sources: Maxim and Delman, 1987; Patel and Cranton, 1983; Tanner, Padrick, Westfall and Pulzier, 1987.

You can see that if you understand the professional processes and the generalizable skills you can use them in any setting in which you work. This is useful when you go to new settings as you can work out what background knowledge you need, what particular skills you need and what services you can offer in that environment so you can prepare yourself beforehand to work in that setting.

BREADTH OR DEPTH OF EXPERIENCE

Previously we talked about the length and number of fieldwork placements and noted that expectations varied considerably depending on your university course. As you go to different placements, you will gain different kinds of experience across a range of services, but the depth of learning in each short placement will necessarily be limited.

There are debates about the optimum range and type of experience that a student should gain before qualifying, and whether emphasis should be placed on depth or breadth of experience. Anderson (1986) claimed that depth of experience across fewer placements encourages deeper understanding and higher levels of competence and enables more sophisticated performance in practice. She argued that anything less should be considered unacceptable. Another way of looking at the debate is to consider the needs of the employer who is trying to serve a specific client group. If, as an employee, you have had more indepth experience with this client group you should be able to meet the needs of these clients more effectively and efficiently than if you have had just one brief encounter on a short fieldwork placement. These would seem to be arguments for fewer, but longer, placements.

In contrast, several shorter placements allow you to see how a number of different organizations function. You meet a number of therapists who work in different ways, and you learn about working with a range of client groups. You gain a more comprehensive view of the profession and of the interrelatedness of institutional and community care. When you consider these points there is still a powerful argument for adhering to the WFOT standards which require breadth in the fieldwork curriculum. This concept also shows how vital it is for newly qualified therapists to have support in the form of adequate supervision and continuing education so that knowledge and skills can be developed as an ongoing process.

Universities normally expect student choice to be built into a curriculum. Students can then decide whether to deepen their understanding of one area of practice or to broaden their knowledge of a range of practices and so keep their employment options open. Having some control over your programme allows you to plan the direction which your learning might take.

SUMMARY

This chapter has explained that professional practice is not static but is constantly evolving and changing to meet different needs and circumstances. Understanding these factors, and being able to adapt to them is vital. Students need to gain an adequate balance of experience in fieldwork education. A limited number of fieldwork placements within an educational programme will never provide the range and level of experience that meet all needs. Students must therefore develop a knowledge and understanding of professional principles and processes and learn to use generalizable skills in new situations. Systems for support and continuing professional education of qualifying therapists are vital for ongoing professional development.

REFERENCES

Anderson, R (1986) Level 11 Fieldwork should become the responsibility of the professional organization. In *Target 2000, Promoting Excellence in Education*. American Occupational Therapy Association, Proceedings from a conference held 22–6 June, 1986.

Fish, D. Twinn, S. and Purr, B. (1991) *Promoting Reflection: Improving the Supervision of Practice in Health Visiting and Initial Teacher Training*. Report Number Two. West London Institute of Higher Education, Twickenham.

Maxim, B. R. and Dielman, T.E. (1987) Dimensionality, internal consistency and interrater reliability of clinical performance ratings. *Medical Education*, **21**, 130–7.

Patel, V. L. and Cranton, P.A. (1983) Transfer of student learning in medical education. *Journal of Medical Education*, **58**, 126–35.

Schon, D. A. (1987) *Educating the Reflective Practitioner*. Jossey-Bass Inc., California.

Tanner, C. A., Padrick, K. P., Westfall, U. A. and Putzier, D. J. (1987) Diagnostic reasoning strategies of nurses and nursing students. *Nursing Research,* []BO]36(6), 358–63.

4 The context of fieldwork

This chapter covers:

- types of settings for fieldwork education;
- constituents of a placement;
- use of non-traditional fieldwork placements;
- elective placements.

Occupational therapists work in many different fields with clients of all ages and with people who have a wide range of problems. This is what makes working in the profession so exciting. Yet each working environment is a unique setting with particular characteristics which together form **the context** of the service provided. Understanding therapy in context is very important as it influences clinical reasoning, professional thinking and ultimately practice. But according to Letts *et al.* (1994) the context of professional practice has not received the same degree of attention as other features of practice. In this chapter we want to explore the qualities of different working environments, and the constituents of fieldwork placements to allow you to make informed decisions about the settings for your fieldwork experience.

SETTINGS OFFERING FIELDWORK PLACEMENTS

Table 4.1 shows the diversity of settings in which occupational therapists work and which have the potential for offering fieldwork placements. The list is quite extensive but not exhaustive. New areas of work are opening up all the time as the profession develops. From the table you can see that occupational therapists are employed in health and social services as well as in education and voluntary services and in private practice. The context of each will be different. Client groups, staffing structures, skill mix and organizational policies and arrangements will affect the context of the work and the kind of fieldwork experience you might have in each setting. It is important that you pay attention to the unique environment of the setting, its peculiarities and limitations, in order to gain a total picture of the way in which services are delivered and the way in which therapists work in that place.

Table 4.1 A selection of health care settings and the services they provide

Setting	*Unit*	*Service*
Hospital	Departments	Accident and emergency Rehabilitation Oncology
	Wards	Acute: medical, surgical, orthopaedic, psychiatric, young physically disabled, elderly
	Specialist services	Eating disorders Stroke Spinal injury Neurological rehabilitation Burns and plastic surgery Behaviour modification Forensic and secure units HIV and AIDS Child and adolescent
	Clinics and day services	Rheumatology Orthopaedic/hand Pain Orthotic and prosthetic Wheelchair and seating Substance abuse Day hospitals for the elderly/respite care Day hospitals for people with mental health problems
Health and social care		Day services for people with mental health problems Day centres for the elderly 'Drop in' and resource centres Refuges
Community	Centres	Primary health care services – doctors' surgeries and health centres Child development centres Community resource centres Disabled living and advisory centres
	Services	Community mental health teams Services for people with learning disabilities
Social services	Departments	Housing and architects
	Teams for:	People with physical disabilities People with mental health problems People recently discharged from hospital Children with special needs Elderly people
Education	Schools	Mainstream Special schools for children with physical and/or learning disabilities
Voluntary sector	Voluntary services	Age Concern MIND Parkinsons' Disease Society SCOPE
Industry	Offices and factories	Occupational health education Pre-retirement programmes
Private	Legal	Medico-legal work and consultancy

BALANCE OF EXPERIENCE IN HOSPITAL AND COMMUNITY SERVICES

Before qualifying as an occupational therapist it is important for you to gain a balance of experience across different hospital and community services and for you to appreciate the interrelationship between them. Considerable emphasis is now placed on the care of clients in the community. Increasingly occupational therapists are taking up posts in the community either as specialist practitioners addressing clients' functional needs, or as care managers assessing needs more generally and purchasing relevant care programmes from others. It has been found (Polatajko, 1994) that functional performance is optimally assessed in the client's occupational context so occupational therapists are ideally suited to working in the community.

You will certainly need to be prepared for community oriented employment when you are qualified. Even if your preference is for hospital-based work, an awareness of the way in which community services are provided will be vital. It will pave the way for effective service delivery across the divides of hospital and community settings, and of health and social care systems, providing a so-called 'seamless service' for clients.

CONSTITUENTS OF A PLACEMENT

The learning opportunities in every placement will be different regardless of whether you are a first year student in your first placement or a final year student in your last placement. The environment, organizational structure, staff team and client group will be unique to that setting and will provide you with a distinctive experience qualitatively different from any other experience you may have.

As we have shown, the list of potential placements is considerable and the experience each placement can offer you is very varied. Identifying common components of a good placement, given the variety of placements, is therefore difficult. There are, however, core elements which should be apparent in any placement and these are shown in Figure 4.1 under the headings: Learning Opportunities, Human Resources, Non-human Resources and The Organization.

Obviously you need access to the service and to clients in order to gain any kind of relevant learning experience. You also need people to guide your practice and other resources to support your fieldwork studies. The way in which the service is organized normally provides the framework in which you work. The efficiency and effectiveness of service organization often has a direct bearing on the quality of fieldwork education you might experience. This is why organizational factors of a placement are often examined as part of an accreditation process. Chapter 6 addresses this further. The accreditation process involves defining standards expected of the fieldwork setting and auditing activity to ensure that standards are operating effectively. It is a quality assurance measure.

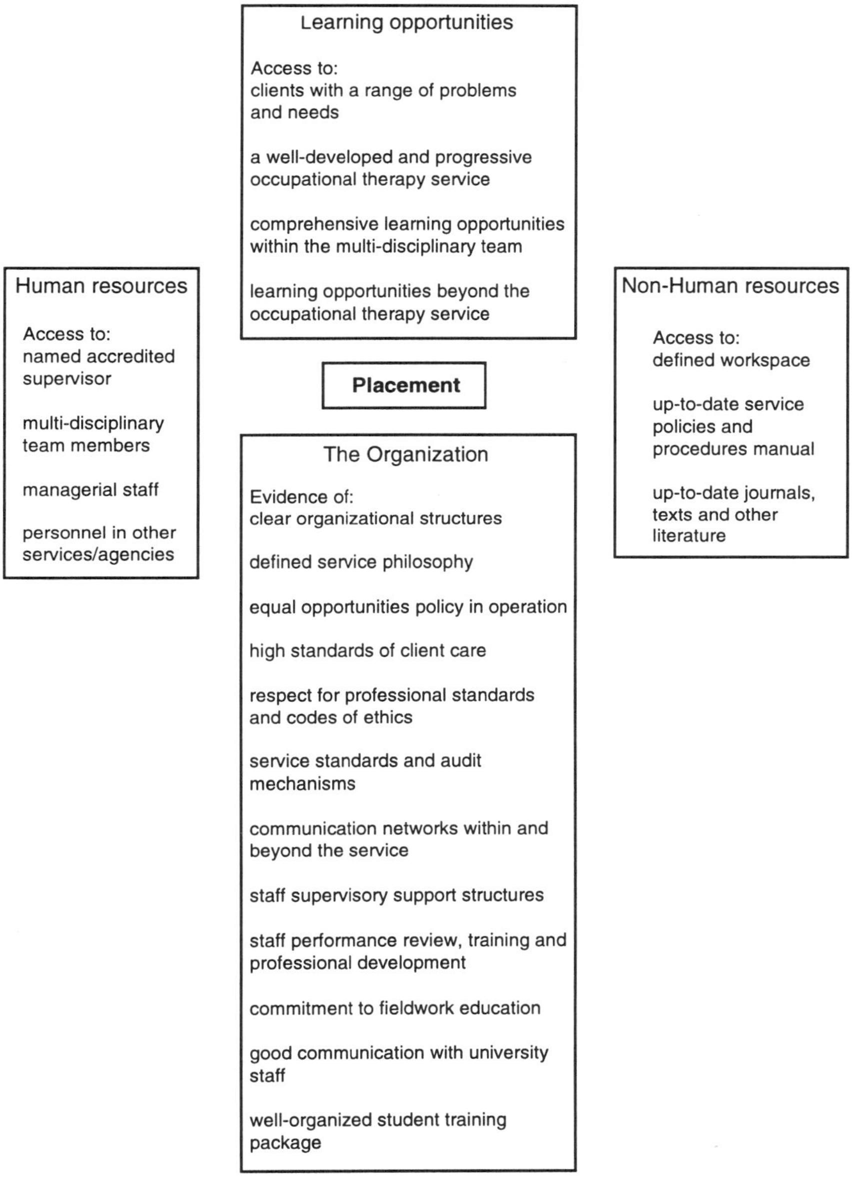

Learning opportunities

Access to:
clients with a range of problems and needs

a well-developed and progressive occupational therapy service

comprehensive learning opportunities within the multi-disciplinary team

learning opportunities beyond the occupational therapy service

Human resources

Access to:
named accredited supervisor

multi-disciplinary team members

managerial staff

personnel in other services/agencies

Placement

Non-Human resources

Access to:
defined workspace

up-to-date service policies and procedures manual

up-to-date journals, texts and other literature

The Organization

Evidence of:
clear organizational structures

defined service philosophy

equal opportunities policy in operation

high standards of client care

respect for professional standards and codes of ethics

service standards and audit mechanisms

communication networks within and beyond the service

staff supervisory support structures

staff performance review, training and professional development

commitment to fieldwork education

good communication with university staff

well-organized student training package

Figure 4.1 Constituents of a placement

STAFF COMMITMENT

Another factor important to the success of a placement is the level of staff commitment to fieldwork education. 'Where there's a will there's a way' is probably one of the most appropriate sayings in our language when it comes to identifying and providing good fieldwork education. Fieldwork educators who really want to offer placements, as opposed to those who are told they have to supervise a student, will usually find a way of providing interesting educational experiences. They will collaborate with university staff and often use innovative problem-solving approaches to overcome any difficulties in arranging fieldwork. They will succeed in creating environments in which effective learning can take place.

PROCEDURES

Clearly, where outcome standards for fieldwork education are defined by the university, fieldwork educators know what structure and processes they need to have in place to assure the quality of fieldwork education. Where standards are explicit it is much easier to identify gaps which need to be filled in order to attain or maintain the standards required. If there are written standards you will know what you can expect of services and of staff with whom you are placed. Where you have a choice of placements, it could well be the quality standards that will influence your decision to accept a placement. Again, we explain this in more detail in Chapter 6.

THE USE OF NON-TRADITIONAL PLACEMENTS

The usual arrangement for fieldwork education is for students to be working and learning under the supervision of an occupational therapist. We have already noted that this is a requirement of programmes recognized by the World Federation of Occupational Therapists. Sometimes, however, it could be in your interest to gain fieldwork experience in a setting in which occupational therapists are not routinely practising and where individuals other than occupational therapists take responsibility for your day to day supervision. In the next paragraphs we explain why this might be so. We also outline the debates about the issue within the profession so that you become aware of the controversy and can make up your own mind about whether such an arrangement might be right for you.

Non-traditional settings

The settings in which non-traditional placements may be offered can be health or social care settings where no occupational therapist is in post but where other healthcare professionals undertake work similar to that normally carried out by occupational therapists. Settings may be those which aim to meet the needs of disabled people in a different way, or the needs of disabled people which are not addressed by statutory services. The settings may therefore be in non-statutory organizations which do not commonly employ occupational therapists. Whatever the arrangement, non-traditional placements are likely to be those which will provide students with very special insights into client needs. An understanding of other perspectives and alternative approaches to meeting needs can serve as a useful foundation for future professional practice.

As we said earlier in the chapter, therapy is increasingly being carried out in the community so that service users can experience 'normal' environments. Examples might include voluntary services for people with mental health problems or problems related to substance abuse, or special clubs, societies or foundations run by, with, or for people with special needs. They might also include community homes for people with dementia, or adults with mental health problems or learning difficulties or services for homeless people.

Non-statutory services and self-help communities frequently operate to a philosophy which promotes enablement and empowerment of service users. Such a philosophy aligns well with the philosophy of Occupational Therapy, a fact highlighted by Stewart (1994). Exposure to such settings would allow you to gain some understanding of the way in which service user needs are identified, prioritized and met according to a value system which might be significantly different to that used in statutory services where a business culture prevails.

Non-traditional placements: debates

You should be aware that there is controversy within the profession about using non-traditional placements, particularly where students do not work under the supervision of an occupational therapist, currently a requirement for insurance purposes. Much concern stems from fears about students not being exposed sufficiently to Occupational Therapy practice to enable their thorough socialization into the profession. Some occupational therapists see these moves as attempts to dilute the profession and to devalue and diminish Occupational Therapy practice. They fear that there will no longer be an Occupational Therapy profession which is uniquely different to other professions if we allow our students to learn their practice from other professionals. They claim that we would be playing into the hands of service managers who are looking to generic or multi-skilled workers to provide client care in a more cost-effective way. It has been suggested, albeit in informal discussion than through empirical study, that other professions use different approaches in their work and do not necessarily use the same, or even a compatible, philosophy. The perception is that students would not be socialized into the profession's unique way of doings things if they worked alongside other professionals, and this would be to the detriment of the student, the client and the profession.

Proposals to use non-traditional settings are not new (AOTA, 1986; Burrows, 1989). Burrows suggested that we should seek to prepare our therapists for the future by maximizing the use of alternative fieldwork settings so that students can gain positive and relevant experiences for future practice. Not everyone shares this vision. The more common perception is that proposals to use non-traditional settings have emerged as a result of difficulties in finding enough placements in Occupational Therapy services for students. If this view alone is propounded it can lead occupational therapists and students into thinking that placements in non-traditional settings might be 'second-rate' alternatives to those in Occupational

Therapy services, rather than positive and beneficial educational experiences in their own right.

We would argue the point that there is nothing wrong with being exposed to other ways of doing things. Leonard Bernstein (1973) the famous conductor, once remarked that a good way of understanding one's own discipline is in the context of another. But some occupational therapists argue that students are not yet mature enough in their professional development to be able to discriminate between the approaches used by different professions and to identify a unique Occupational Therapy way of working. It is sometimes suggested that students early in their career are not yet clear about the specifics of Occupational Therapy and that they need as much exposure as possible to the profession to gain insights into the way in which occupational therapists work.

Core skills and values

Another argument against non-traditional settings is that students need to gain a strong identity with their own profession and a strong sense of the profession's core skills and values before qualifying. It is argued that students need as much practice as possible in applying profession specific skills and evaluating practice under the supervision of an occupational therapist who acts as a role model in the workplace. According to Swinehart and Mayers (1993) students need help to assess and analyse problems in a profession-specific way and to understand, draw on and use profession-specific theories to underpin professional practice before they gain experience of working with other professionals. Clearly we cannot argue against the need for students to acquire the profession's core skills and values if we wish to see competent and confident occupational therapists emerge on qualification to take their place in the profession and move it forward. Equally, however, Occupational Therapy students need to learn from the outset how to work with other professionals in teams and to be able to both distinguish and integrate profession-specific skills in practice.

Generic therapists

Another facet of this continuing debate on the use of non-traditional placements is that of the training and use of generic therapists or multi-skilled workers. It is foreseen that such people will have a general grounding in rehabilitation principles which are drawn from several professions. The threats of these emerging generic and multi-skilled workers are very real to occupational therapists whose jobs are at stake and who are being required to work in a very different way. Their protection of a profession which they hold dear is not in itself surprising as they resist any attempt to expose students to alternative practices which might encourage the development of generic worker skills. It is worth noting, however, that there is another argument which suggests that the employment of generic therapists frees up more highly qualified occupational therapists to plan service programmes, educate the team and develop research opportunities.

Stereotyping students

What is surprising, however, is the stereotyping of students which emerges as views about non-traditional placements are expressed. In its practice, the Occupational Therapy profession claims to acknowledge each person as an individual, with different strengths, limitations and needs. The same philosophy can be applied to the student population. Occupational Therapy students come in all sorts of shapes and sizes, from different backgrounds and with different life experiences. So it is not clear why assumptions should automatically be made that every student regardless of background should need exactly the same exposure to Occupational Therapy practice as every other student in order to become a competent practitioner. If we were to assess strengths and needs, and provide a programme to suit, then the type of experiences and the number of hours spent in fieldwork would vary from student to student. The input, ie the services to which the student is exposed and the number of hours required for qualification, would be modified accordingly. Whatever the input, the responsibility would be on the student to demonstrate competence to practise as the desired outcome of professional education.

Many Occupational Therapy students these days have worked in an Occupational Therapy service and have gained insights into professional practice prior to entry to the course. Many are mature in their outlook and already have the capacity to be able to distinguish between different approaches to care provision. They are able to appreciate good practice regardless of the profession to which the individual belongs (Alsop, 1991). They can select and, if necessary, reject elements of practice for their own repertoire according to their own value system. Equally there are other students who find this more difficult early in their programme of education. There is nothing wrong with that at all. Some students just need more guidance to come to terms with the core skills, processes and approaches used by the profession through exposure directly to Occupational Therapy practice. If this is either the perceived or the expressed need, it should be met.

Shortage of placements

It is true that for some time now there has been a shortage of placements for Occupational Therapy students, reported in other countries and not just the UK (Tompson and Tompson 1987). Professions such as social work have been experiencing the same difficulty (Hepstinall, 1987; Pottinger, 1988). Numbers of students needing placements have increased at a time when organizational changes within the health and social care system have been taking place. For instance, large psychiatric hospitals which formerly provided a significant number of student placements at any one time, have been closing. More occupational therapists now work independently, rather than in large departments, or work as members of multi-disciplinary or inter-disciplinary teams. They do not have the support systems that were previously in place in hospitals. Community services provide very relevant learning experiences for students as preparation for future employment, but the number of students able to access the new services is considerably reduced since rationalization and changes in modes of service delivery.

Similarly, in Local Authorities reorganization of services in line with government reforms made it difficult for occupational therapists to manage both the reforms and student placements at the same time, so the provision of placements was suspended. The loss of many placements all at once challenged the profession to be more liberal in its thinking about what might constitute suitable alternative learning experiences for students which would not threaten professional standards. These trends also reinforce our assertion that students need to develop the ability to act autonomously, work creatively and show resourcefulness in practice and thus need experience which is going to help develop these qualities.

Some Occupational Therapy programmes in the UK have initiated a range of small-scale schemes to provide placements for students in non-traditional settings for short periods of time. But often the hours in services where there is no occupational therapist can not be counted towards the 1000 hours required for professional qualification even though they might provide very relevant learning experiences. Research is perhaps needed into what might be justifiably regarded as relevant learning experiences.

The requirement for students to work directly under the supervision of an occupational therapist has limited the development of larger-scale initiatives which could provide suitable learning opportunities and help prepare students to work independently once qualified. Given commitment, sound preparation and a well-developed infra-structure to support placements there is no reason why alternative strategies for providing fieldwork experience should not be developed. Criteria for such initiatives are proposed shortly. The *Guidelines* from the College of Occupational Therapists (1993) authorize models of student supervision which should allow for more creativity in developing schemes for fieldwork education.

Successful schemes in the United States of America established legitimately for Level One Fieldwork provide examples of placements where students are able to observe and participate in fieldwork under the supervision of personnel such as teachers, social workers, ministers, probation officers, nurses and physical therapists (Kautzmann, 1987). Not all are successful as Swinehart and Meyers (1993) point out. However, it is these sort of initiatives that need to be carefully implemented, monitored, evaluated and developed with a view to increasing the range of satisfactory learning opportunities for students in the future.

These are some of the current debates about using non-traditional placements. It is true that non-traditional placements are sometimes seen as a back-up or even a last resort for when placements of the more traditional kind are not available. But this is not an educationally sound practice. Non-traditional placements should only be used when the aims and objectives for fieldwork education for a particular student are clear and can be met in that placement.

Advantages of using non-traditional placements

We suggest that non-traditional placements may have the following clear advantages and should sometimes be favoured instead of placements in traditional Occupational Therapy services.

- You might gain experience in an area where occupational therapists might come to practise more routinely in the future. This is how the profession advances into new and developing areas.

- You might gain experience with clients for whom Occupational Therapy is not readily available. This may be because of lack of funds to support a post, because of a 'frozen' post, because of an inability to recruit, because another professional is doing a job which might equally be done by an occupational therapist, or because no one has yet recognized the need for Occupational Therapy provision.
- You might be exposed to alternative approaches to care and/or alternative professional perspectives and so enhance your overall understanding of care provision,
- You might gain relevant skills to complement those already in your repertoire, but which need not necessarily be taught by an occupational therapist,
- You might gain more varied work experience and more broad-based learning as preparation for future practice.

A secondary gain could be that non-occupational therapists become better informed about Occupational Therapy practice so improving inter-professional working relationships.

Ensuring the effectiveness of non-traditional placements

Obviously for the placement to be accepted it must meet the course objectives and your specific learning needs. For the placement to be effective it is critical that an appropriate structure be established to support it. As a bare minimum there will need to be:

- an acceptance by both you and the university of the potential of the placement and confirmation of appropriate insurance cover;
- a willingness of the designated fieldwork educator to accept the responsibilities of the role, and to undertake any training for that role;
- a designated experienced occupational therapist to support you, to collaborate with the day-to-day educator and to assess you on the Occupational Therapy-specific components of practice; this person could be your academic tutor at university;
- clear definitions of roles, rights and responsibilities of the parties involved;
- excellent communication between course staff and the fieldwork educators;
- explicit support mechanisms for you and your educator and a clear procedure for managing difficulties should they arise;
- an individually tailored programme which reflects your learning needs and the placement objectives.

We come back to our saying 'where there's a will there's a way' in relation to non-traditional placements. It is unlikely ever to be the norm for all students of Occupational Therapy to undertake a placement in a non-traditional setting. We cannot foresee circumstances in which students would ever undertake more than one non-traditional placement during their qualifying programme. But there is no doubt that very occasionally a non-traditional setting could well provide an excellent learning environment. Opportunities such as these should be nurtured and used in the most constructive way.

ACCEPTING A PLACEMENT

When placements are arranged by university staff, your previous experience and preferred way of working is normally taken into consideration. Hopefully you will have some choice about the context in which you gain your fieldwork experience. You must ask about insurance cover. You might also ask about standards and whether accreditation systems are in place. You might wish to influence the decision about your placements. It is up to you to make your views known about whether you might be prepared to undertake a fieldwork placement in a non-traditional setting. But remember, there is no obligation for you to accept such a placement if one is offered, particularly where the support mechanisms might be weak. Do check this out. The above criteria for an effective fieldwork placement might guide your questions.

ELECTIVE PLACEMENTS

In some educational programmes students are given the opportunity to undertake an **elective** placement, that is a placement of your own choice which you arrange for yourself. Elective placements provide students with opportunities to develop personal interests related to Occupational Therapy practice either within or beyond the usual Occupational Therapy services. Some students apply to more specialist areas of Occupational Therapy practice, others venture abroad to gain experience of health care systems in other countries. Supervision may be arranged, for instance, with a fully accredited fieldwork educator in the host country or perhaps with an occupational therapist working in such organizations as the Voluntary Services Overseas (VSO). There are many possibilities. For some placements there may be no direct supervision from an occupational therapist. Arrangements will be made with a relevant named person who can provide support, supervision and some evaluation of practice.

The exact criteria for elective placements are established by the University. There may be conditions about whether the hours worked in elective placements are supplementary to the 1000 hours needed for qualifying, and whether the elective placement must be undertaken under the supervision of an occupational therapist. Whatever the conditions imposed, an elective placement will offer you a one-off opportunity to gain a very different kind of experience while still operating as a student, with the relative security that status affords. You also have the responsibility for organizing the placement yourself, and that can help develop your management skills.

If you are going abroad you need to make special arrangements for insurance and health protection, to be clear about the support mechanisms in place and about who will be assessing your performance. Provided that the elective placement is well-planned, you will almost certainly return to university having achieved considerable personal and professional growth and broadened your understanding of different approaches to health care provision.

SUMMARY

In this chapter we have examined the kinds of settings, both traditional and non-traditional, that you might access as a student, and we have explored some of the debates about using non-traditional placements. We have advocated that it is desirable for you to gain some experience in a community setting as preparation for practice once you are qualified. Whatever the opportunities available to you, the placement should allow you to develop the skills and qualities needed for independent practice and give you a clear understanding of the unique contribution that occupational therapists bring to client care.

REFERENCES

Alsop, A. (1991) *Five Schools Project: Clinical Practice Curriculum Development.* Unpublished report, Dorset House School of Occupational Therapy, Oxford.

AOTA (1986) *Target 2000: Promoting Excellence in Education.* Conference Proceedings, 22–6 June, American Occupational Therapy Association, Rockville MD.

Bernstein, L. (1973) Norton Lectures at Harvard, presented on BBC Television, December 1990.

Burrows, E. (1989) Maximising clinical practice. Editorial. *British Journal of Occupational Therapy*, **52**(2), 41.

College of Occupational Therapists (1993) *Guidelines for Assuring the Quality of Fieldwork Education of Occupational Therapy Students.* SPP165, College of Occupational Therapists, London.

Hepstinall, D. (1987) The placement shortfall. *Social Services Insight,* 21 August 1987.

Kautzmann, L. N. (1987) Perceptions of the purpose of Level 1 fieldwork. *American Journal of Occupational Therapy*, **41**, 595–600.

Letts, L., Law, M., Rigby, P., Cooper, B., Stewart, D. and Strong, S. (1994) Person-environment assessments in occupational therapy. *American Journal of Occupational Therapy*, **48**(7), 595–607.

Polatajko, H. (1994) Dreams, dilemmas and decisions for occupational therapy practice in the new millennium: a Canadian perspective. *American Journal of Occupational Therapy*, **48**(7), 590–94.

Pottinger, J. (1988) The practice placement crisis, accreditation and joint appointments. *Social Work Today*, **7**(2), 29–30.

Stewart, A. (1994) Empowerment and enablement: occupational therapy 2001. *British Journal of Occupational Therapy*, **57**(7), 248–54.

Swinehart, S. and Meyers, S. K. (1993) Level 1 Fieldwork: creating a positive experience. *American Journal of Occupational Therapy*, **47**(1), 68–73.

Tompson, M. A. and Tompson, C. (1987) The Canadian approach to fieldwork. *Canadian Journal of Occupational Therapy*, **54**(5), 243–8.

5 Allocation of placements

This chapter covers:

- the management of fieldwork education;
- the fieldwork placement prospectus;
- the allocation of fieldwork placements;
- students with special needs

This chapter is intended to give you some background information about placement allocation and the kind of preparations that need to be made prior to fieldwork education.

The allocation of fieldwork placements is a very complex task particularly for courses which have large numbers of students. Finding sufficient good quality placements is not easy. There are two main reasons. Firstly, placements are not plentiful, there are barely enough placements nationally to meet all student needs. Secondly, there is no obligation for services to offer placements, or to provide placements of adequate quality. Much depends on good will and on good working relationships existing between academic and fieldwork staff.

The College of Occupational Therapists (1995) sees it as a moral and professional responsibility for clinicians to provide opportunities for students to gain the experience they need for professional qualification. The NHS Management Executive also expects services to provide placements to ensure that adequate numbers of suitably qualified personnel are trained for work in the NHS. Availability of placements ultimately depends on individual services' willingness to accept students for training, and on satisfactory staffing levels to cope with the workload.

MANAGING FIELDWORK EDUCATION

A member of the university staff usually known as the fieldwork coordinator takes prime responsibility for the overall management of fieldwork education, and that person will take steps to locate suitable placements. Sometimes this means approaching fieldwork settings directly and offering to support staff who have shown an interest in becoming fieldwork educators. Alternatively a therapist may approach the university and indicate a willingness to educate students and offer placements. The fieldwork coordinator will visit the service and discuss the provision of fieldwork education in the new setting. He or she will explain course requirements and fieldwork objectives and ensure that the clinician has the skills to educate students and to manage their placement effectively. The fieldwork coordinator will also implement any accreditation procedure on behalf of the university and will normally make the ultimate judgement about the suitability of a placement for student education. A fieldwork manual which contains information about the course and its assessment requirements is usually made available to fieldwork educators.

THE PLACEMENT PROSPECTUS

Fieldwork educators are asked to provide an information pack, or better still a prospectus, detailing what the placement has to offer, to be kept at the university for consultation. The following is the sort of information which might be found in a prospectus:

- location of the placement/map;
- description of the facilities;
- relationship of the Occupational Therapy service within the wider organization;
- mode of service provision;
- service philosophy and mission statement;
- models and/or approaches used by occupational therapists and other team members;
- nature of the client group;
- staffing arrangements;
- staffing expertise;
- nature of the student experience both within and beyond the fieldwork setting;
- learning opportunities and educational experiences on offer;
- criteria to be met for accessing the placement;
- contractual arrangements;
- availability of accommodation;
- name and telephone number of contact for further information.

Information packs sometimes contain other relevant information such as a more detailed profile of the Occupational Therapy service and information on local leisure facilities and transport services.

PLACEMENT ALLOCATION

The task of allocating placements normally falls to the university. Some universities have computerized systems to assist with the process, others prefer to rely on manual systems of allocation. Some countries, such as Canada, have a national computerized system for this purpose. Allocating placements using a computerized system has many advantages. From the data that is stored on computer, information about a student's fieldwork experience throughout his or her course can be retrieved. The frequency of using a particular placement over time can also be tracked, and spare capacity within the system can be readily identified.

For the process of placement allocation, some universities identify available placements and then allocate students to them, making sure that each student gains a balance of experience overall. Other universities start by examining a student's previous experience and identify appropriate placements to ensure balanced experience across different fields of Occupational Therapy. Sometimes students plan their own fieldwork education programme using criteria and information about placements supplied by the university. The fieldwork coordinator monitors the process to ensure that placements do not get double-booked.

ALLOCATING PLACEMENTS FAIRLY

Allocation has to take account of placement availability and every student's needs. Your cooperation, patience and tolerance are therefore essential when placements are allocated. Everyone has to be catered for fairly. You may be offered choice but ultimately students have to be matched to the placements available. Sometimes student demand and placement availability do not match. There may be times when you will need to be flexible about the placements you accept, and there may be times when your particular preferences for placements cannot be given. 'Give and take' in the allocation process is expected of everyone.

PLACEMENT SHORTAGES AND CANCELLATIONS

We have already alerted you to the difficulties experienced in finding placements. Apart from changes within a service there are other reasons why placement shortages may occur. Temporary difficulties sometimes arise due to inadequate staffing levels caused by staff vacancies, maternity leave, sick leave, study leave and so on. As staffing levels fluctuate so does the availability of placements. Placement provision is beyond the control of the university and placements can be withdrawn for all sorts of reasons. Even if placements have previously been agreed and allocated, cancellation can occur at the last moment. All cancellations create extra work for the fieldwork coordinator, and anxiety for the student concerned.

Fieldwork educators, as clinicians, are under enormous pressures and a small change in circumstances at work can prompt them to cancel the placement. Fieldwork educators may not always appreciate the difficulty caused by last minute cancellations and the upset this causes to students. Students may have made extensive adjustments in their life to undertake the placement, particularly if it means staying away from home. It can mean a total revision of plans which impinge on personal as well as academic life.

Any cancellation means that another service has to be approached at very short notice for a placement and, when found, everyone must work to very tight schedules to prepare for the fieldwork experience. There may even be times when a placement has to be deferred if the schedules cannot be met. This is not ideal, but it may be a better option than commencing a placement which is not sufficiently prepared.

Difficulties within an Occupational Therapy service do not automatically mean that placements are cancelled. Sometimes the placement can proceed after a review of the circumstances and the level of support available to the student. Fieldwork educators can be very accommodating and often find ways to adjust the placement so as to make it viable. Many educators find creative ways of managing both the problem and the student successfully. If the placement goes ahead, the type of experience a student receives may not be as originally intended but it can be an equally successful placement. Students do need to be realistic in their expectations of fieldwork placements and be tolerant if a placement has to be changed. Difficulties arising from placement cancellations have to be managed as best they can.

SPECIAL NEEDS

Whatever the process of allocating placements, any special needs that you have will normally be taken into consideration. These may be special needs relating to health-related matters or to personal circumstances. It is quite possible, for instance, for students to have a sight or hearing impairment, back problems, or to suffer from conditions such as epilepsy or diabetes mellitus, or other conditions which need special consideration. None of these need interfere with fieldwork education provided that needs are discussed with the fieldwork coordinator and fieldwork educator and steps are taken to minimize any forseeable risks.

THE FIELDWORK EDUCATION AGREEMENT

Once placements have been allocated, they are confirmed by letter and sometimes more formally with a placement contract. The fieldwork education agreement, or placement contract, is a formal agreement between the service and the university which sets out the terms and conditions of the placement and specifies the expectations and responsibilities of each party to the agreement.

Within the agreement statements may be made about:

- availability and competence of staff;
- characteristics of supervision;
- student competence and conduct;
- the preparation of students for the placement;
- student support;
- student assessment;
- placement monitoring and feedback;
- organizational policies and procedures;
- access to libraries and other resources;

- insurance and indemnity;
- reimbursement of expenses.

A more formal agreement clarifies expectations and acts as a quality monitoring mechanism for fieldwork education. If there is a breach of the agreement by the service the student may be withdrawn from the placement, if there is a breach in the agreement by the university the service may withdraw the placement.

COMMUNICATION BETWEEN THE UNIVERSITY AND FIELDWORK SETTING

Regardless of any formal agreement there does need to be some written communication between the university and the service to confirm the fieldwork arrangements. As the placement approaches, and normally within six weeks of its commencement, the university should confirm details of the placement and provide the service with the names of the students. Communication can then be initiated between the fieldwork educator and the student and final preparations for the placement can be made. These preparations and other practical arrangements are discussed in Chapter 9.

SUMMARY

This chapter has explained how placements are managed and allocated to ensure that students gain a balance of fieldwork experiences as part of their educational programme. Difficulties in the system have been highlighted. Although every effort is made to ensure a satisfactory fieldwork experience there are times when the allocation process does not go according to plan and cancellations occur. Students are encouraged to be cooperative and tolerant in times of difficulty and need to be prepared to accept alternative options for placements.

REFERENCES

Code of Ethics and Professional Conduct for Occupational Therapists (1995) College of Occupational Therapists, London.

Falk-Kessler, J., Barnowski, C. and Salvant, S. (1994) Mandatory HIV testing and Occupational Therapists. *American Journal of Occupational Therapy*, **48**(1), 27–37.

Accreditation and qualities of the fieldwork educator

6

This chapter covers:

- accreditation systems and processes;
- characteristics of the fieldwork educator;
- preparation of fieldwork educators for their role;
- models of educational relationships between student and fieldwork educator.

When you entered university you no doubt expected your lecturers to be well qualified in their specialist field and to have the necessary skills and qualifications to teach in the academic setting. It is not unusual for occupational therapists who become university lecturers to have, or to be working towards, a Master's degree and increasingly frequently nowadays, a PhD. New lecturers who have no formal teaching qualification are also normally required by the university to study for a post graduate certificate in higher education (PGCHE). The aim is to ensure that those responsible for your education are properly qualified.

When you go on placement, your expectations of the fieldwork educators may be exactly the same – that they are well qualified in their specialist field and that they have the necessary skills and qualifications to teach in the fieldwork setting. But the emphasis in the fieldwork setting is somewhat different to that of the academic setting because the primary role of a fieldwork educator is that of a practitioner. Being an educator is a secondary role. The practitioner is employed, not by the university but by a service to deliver client care and for this reason greater emphasis tends to be placed on the continuing development of the practitioner's clinical competence and skills than on the accumulation of educational qualifications.

Nevertheless, fieldwork education is an educational process. Those who extend their clinical role to become fieldwork educators are thus expected to develop their knowledge of adult educational processes. They also need to be able to manage fieldwork in addition to their other responsibilities. Fieldwork educator programmes are often organized by universities to prepare educators for their extended role. This preparation may lead to practitioners becoming accredited as fieldwork educators by the university. Accreditation acknowledges the practitioner's proven ability to act as a fieldwork educator and his or her readiness to comply with requirements of the role.

ACCREDITATION

Quality assurance mechanisms are established to make explicit the standard of performance which can be expected by consumers of those delivering a service to them. Accreditation is the formal process of auditing those standards by a body empowered to judge and certify that the standards have been achieved. Accreditation is both a quality assurance process and the recognition given for having met pre-determined criteria.

Sometimes confusion arises about the meaning of the word accreditation. In the UK, the College of Occupational Therapists expects Occupational Therapy programmes in universities to accredit fieldwork placements and/or fieldwork educators. The College of Occupational Therapists (1994) defines accreditation as 'the formal process whereby the education centre recognises good practice' (p. 4). In the UK there is a distinction made between **validation** and **accreditation**. Educational programmes designed and written by the university are **validated** which means that they are approved to run. Individuals qualifying from Occupational Therapy programmes which have also been validated by the profession are eligible for State Registration. In other countries this process is known as accreditation. In the United States only graduates who complete an accredited [validated] programme are eligible to sit for the American Occupational Therapy Registration Board examination to become an Occupational Therapist Registered (OTR) (Graves, 1994). In Canada, Occupational Therapy students must complete a minimum number of 1000 hours in accredited fieldwork sites before graduation, and a national body has responsibility for accreditation of the placements (Christiansen and Christiansen 1994). For ease of reference, the terms used in the UK will be those used throughout this book.

PURPOSE AND PROCESS OF ACCREDITATION

The College of Occupational Therapists (1994) has guidelines detailing the expectations it has of those accredited to act as fieldwork educators. The guidelines are implemented by universities which ensure that educators are trained to meet the standards and expectations of the profession. Universities operate flexible systems to enable practitioners to become accredited as fieldwork educators. Practitioners may participate in a fieldwork educator programme with other practitioners. Alternatively they may elect to work independently and prepare a portfolio which is then assessed by the university to determine the practitioner's ability to educate students.

Accreditation of fieldwork placements and fieldwork educators

There is continuing professional debate about whether fieldwork placements or fieldwork educators should be accredited, or both. There are arguments for both systems. One line of thought is that the context in which fieldwork education is provided is important and that an accreditation process should examine the fieldwork environment and not just the practitioners involved. The other line of thought is that practitioners, once they have developed and demonstrated the required knowledge, skills and attitudes to educate students, should be accredited as fieldwork educators by the university. Accredited fieldwork educators should then take the responsibility for ensuring that the quality of the fieldwork experience provided for students is satisfactory.

ACCREDITATION OF PLACEMENTS

The College of Occupational Therapists (1991) originally recommended standards for the management of fieldwork education which included statements on service organization and management. Some Occupational Therapy programmes established their accreditation systems around these standards. Occupational Therapy services which offered placements and which sought accreditation were then audited. Those which met the standards were accredited. This procedure takes time to complete and there are resource implications. It is also acknowledged that accreditation can only reflect the way in which the service is operating on the day of the accreditation. In 1993 the COT withdrew these recommendations and subsequently approved new guidelines for the Accreditation of Fieldwork Educators (College of Occupational Therapists, 1994). Some universities continue to operate accreditation systems in line with the earlier requirements.

ACCREDITATION OF FIELDWORK EDUCATORS

The accreditation of fieldwork educators is slightly different. This process relies on the individual acquiring relevant knowledge, skills and attitudes for the effective delivery of fieldwork education. It relies on the fieldwork educator developing the ability to make an informed decision about the suitability of a placement. He or she must be able to discriminate between good and bad learning opportunities and make judgements about a placement regardless of the setting. He or she will assess the merits of providing student placements on behalf of the university and will know how to improve the environment where necessary so that placements can be offered. The education and development of fieldwork educators to a very high standard is thus crucial to the development and retention of good quality placements. In the current climate of rapid change this seems a more achievable and workable system.

CHARACTERISTICS OF A FIELDWORK EDUCATOR

Wallis (1987) argues that one of the expectations of a professional is that he or she should participate in the training of learners and junior members of the profession, and should strive to advance the field in which he or she is practising. But not all practitioners want to become fieldwork educators even though it might be considered a professional responsibility. According to students, not all good practitioners make good fieldwork educators (Alsop, 1991) so perhaps those who feel less inclined to take on this responsibility should not be forced to do so. Practitioners may have excellent therapeutic skills but the problem seems to lie in their ability to communicate these skills to students. Edwards and Baptiste (1987) state that:

> an assumption is made that the clinicians have the necessary skills to facilitate the learners, accurately grade their performance and provide effective feedback. While clinicians may possess excellent clinical skills and be appropriate role models for students, additional or adapted skills are often required to assess clinical competence (p. 249).

Alsop's (1991) study proposed that a practitioner needs to develop interpersonal, supervisory and managerial skills in order to act effectively as a fieldwork educator. From this it was argued that fieldwork educators need to:

1. practise as a competent practitioner;
2. be able to manage themselves and the student in the workplace;
3. know how to teach students, and guide and facilitate their learning;
4. know how to support students during their placement;
5. know how to evaluate students' performance and assess their competence to practise.

It is these requirements that form the basis of the College of Occupational Therapists' (1994) guidelines for the accreditation of fieldwork educators. An explanation is given below.

1. Practising as a competent practitioner

The first characteristic of a fieldwork educator is that he or she performs competently and confidently as a practitioner. Integral to competence is a requirement that the practitioner practises legally, ethically and in a non-judgemental, non-discriminatory way. The practitioner must have the ability to reflect on, and evaluate, his or her own practice and learn from those reflections as a pre-requisite to evaluating the practice of students. The practitioner must also be able to use sound clinical reasoning skills in the execution of duties with clients.

Not only is it important for practitioners wishing to become fieldwork educators to have knowledge, skills and expertise in their own field, they must also be committed to the education of students. It is important that the decision to become a fieldwork educator is freely made, even if the decision is made as a result of prompting by the line manager. Occasionally practitioners are required, because of their job description or service standards, to engage in student education but feel uncomfortable with these responsibilities. Such demands can create tensions in the relationship with students. Whenever the decision is made for a clinician to become a fieldwork educator it is crucial that the individual has support and supervision from his or her line manager when the additional responsibilities are assumed.

2. Performing as a manager

Before taking responsibility for a student, a fieldwork educator must first demonstrate competence as a manager of his or her own situation. This will include not only the ability to manage a caseload but also to manage other resources, for instance time, or other staff under his or her supervision, and to manage other duties and responsibilities that he or she has to fulfil in the workplace. Only then can the practitioner accept responsibility for planning, directing, implementing, monitoring and evaluating, in other words managing, a student's experience.

Managing a student's placement is quite a complex task. The fieldwork educator must liaise with the university and gain an understanding of the fieldwork curriculum and implement it. He or she must also take decisions about the suitability of the learning environment for fieldwork education, prepare colleagues and team members for the student's arrival, plan the student's programme and manage any difficulties or conflicts arising during the placement. The fieldwork educator may be responsible for agreeing the placement contract with the university, for negotiating the learning contract with the student, for ensuring that the student is briefed in health and safety requirements and for allocating responsibilities regarding client care. Regardless of managing all tasks relating to the fieldwork placement, the practitioner still has primary responsibility for managing client care.

At the beginning of the placement the fieldwork educator must ensure that the student is properly briefed about his or her role, particularly in relation to legal requirements. During the placement the fieldwork educator has to monitor the student's progress and has to ensure that he or she fulfils the expectations of the university in respect of the fieldwork experience. At the end of the placement the fieldwork educator has to ensure that the student's withdrawal from the placement is managed effectively.

3. Enabling learning

Being an educator involves enabling students to become actively involved in the learning process as a journey of discovery. This demands very high levels of skill on the part of the fieldwork educator. It is crucial to the whole fieldwork experience that the fieldwork educator engages in the process of **educating** rather than merely supervising students and **facilitates learning** through reflection on practice.

Being an enabler of learning also entails knowing about those factors which can either facilitate or impede learning, for instance, differences in learning styles. It is also important for the educator to have a clear idea about the meaning of the learning experience to the learner. The educator must therefore have a working knowledge of adult education theories, of theories of motivation, clinical reasoning concepts and of theories relating to stages of student development. Knowledge of student development is necessary for understanding students' needs and expectations as each person may operate at a different conceptual level. The fieldwork educator has to be conversant with these theories so that he or she can identify the stage at which a student is operating and select appropriate strategies for moving the student to the next stage of development.

4. Counselling and supporting students

There may be times during the fieldwork experience when students need extra help, support or advice about a matter either to do with learning or to do with something personal. Problems may adversely affect behaviour or performance so it is important that needs and problems are addressed.

There can be a conflict of roles for someone who not only has to guide learning and assess performance, but who also has to act as an advisor, supporter or counsellor in the process. But since learning will only take place if an individual is receptive to it, anything that interferes with learning needs to be addressed. It should be noted, however, that there is a considerable difference between someone who uses counselling skills and someone who acts as a counsellor (Burnard, 1994). Counsellors have had specialist training and have qualifications in addition to profession specific qualifications and will know how and when to draw on specialist techniques for counselling. A fieldwork educator might be perceived to have counselling skills because of his or her role with clients, but it is important for the educator to be able to distinguish between a therapeutic and an educational relationship and not to confuse the two in the process of working with the student. One of the most important skills of a fieldwork educator is therefore to recognize the limits of his or her ability and to know when to refer a student to another source for further help.

5. Assessing and evaluating performance

This is a crucial responsibility for the fieldwork educator. Ilott (1995) suggests that a fieldwork educator is 'a gatekeeper of the profession' in assessing a student's competence to practise. But it is necessary to remember that the fieldwork educator has also been involved in trying to develop that competence and some would argue that it is very difficult to combine both the roles of educator and assessor satisfactorily. Often it is recommended that the two functions remain separated, but in fieldwork education they are combined.

The educator must have the skills to judge competent performance and to be able to test and probe knowledge in order to verify a student's competence. The educator must be conversant with the particular assessment or evaluation form used by the university and understand the grading system. Lastly, a fieldwork educator must be able to take responsibility for failing a student where this is judged to be the right course of action. Failing a student is never an easy thing to cope with either for the student or the educator (Ilott, 1995) but since the educator has a responsibility to the public and to the profession only to allow competent individuals to qualify, the educator must have the confidence and competence to make this judgement and carry it through.

PREPARING FIELDWORK EDUCATORS FOR THEIR ROLE

The development of the fieldwork educator's skills beyond that of a competent practitioner is essential for effective student education and only when these skills have been developed to a reasonable standard should accreditation be awarded. It is likely to take time for a practitioner to develop those skills so an interim arrangement would be for a university to approve a practitioner as a fieldwork educator so that he or she can become involved in the process of student education and start to develop the skills needed for accreditation. Figure 6.1 illustrates one route that may be followed.

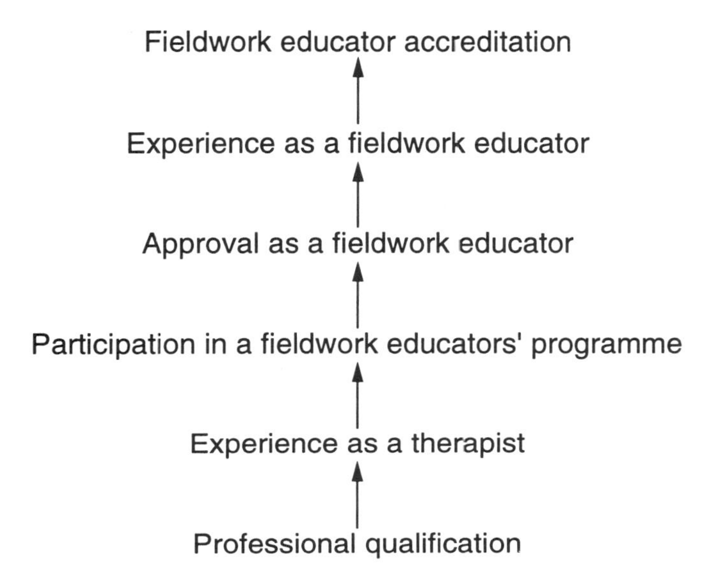

Figure 6.1 Accreditation and qualities of the fieldwork educator

The fieldwork educator will learn from the experience of educating students and from engaging with the student in the process of reflection. As a student, you may be involved in some of the reflective discussions as the fieldwork educator seeks feedback from you about his or her performance as an educator. Fieldwork education thus becomes a two way process of learning.

There is general agreement within the profession that practitioners need to be educated and prepared for this role but the extent of this preparation is open to interpretation. Clinical supervisor courses formerly approved by the College of Occupational Therapists, albeit effective, tended to concentrate on the more procedural aspects of managing the placement and provided only limited input on educational theories which underpin the fieldwork experience. The result was that supervisors acted as models for students, teaching them rather than facilitating their learning, and students often 'got by' on the placement because the supervisor was reluctant to fail them. Both the profession and the university now have greater expectations of fieldwork educators, most particularly that they will be educators.

Practitioners committed to the education of students will be motivated to develop appropriate skills, but the majority expect to be able to attend relevant courses during working hours. Although fieldwork educator programmes help structure and promote skill development, many of the skills needed by educators can only really be developed through practice. A minority of practitioners, however, see no reason to develop their skills at all. They perceive that educating students is a simple extension of their role as therapists and that knowledge of principles of teaching learnt during their qualifying programme is sufficient preparation for the role of educator.

Educational programmes shared with other professions

Professions such as physiotherapy, nursing and social work each specify the way in which their members should prepare for their role as student educators. More recently programmes have been devised which involve shared learning between the professions since many of the skills needed to educate and assess students are considered to be similar regardless of the professional background. However, these programmes have been found to be very time-consuming to organize because time first has to be spent in clarifying the different professional perspectives and in ensuring that the needs of all the professions represented are integrated into the shared programme. But there are advantages in using shared learning opportunities. Many students have placements in multi- or inter-disciplinary teams where several members can be involved in the educational process. Members of other professions now manage some of the day-to-day elements of a fieldwork placement. Educators can be better prepared for their role if preparation is undertaken alongside members of other professions.

Personal attributes of fieldwork educators

This chapter has highlighted the extent to which fieldwork educators need to develop attitudes, knowledge and additional skills to fulfil their role effectively. Interactive skills also need to be developed as they are perceived by students to be crucial to the supervisory relationship. We list in Table 6.1 some of the personal attributes found in fieldwork educators which have been identified in researched findings (Christie *et al.*, 1985; Kautzmann, 1990). They are not listed in any special order of priority but you will find that they are consistent with the five key areas of skill development described above.

We hope you do not experience any of the negative attitudes during your fieldwork experience, but if you do, try to think about why these attitudes prevail and what you might do about them. Alsop's (1991) report suggested that student learning was affected quite significantly when negative attitudes prevailed as Table 6.2 shows, so it is important that these negative attitudes are not allowed to dominate the learning experience.

Table 6.3 shows how meaningful learning can result from students having positive experiences during their fieldwork education. You can see, then, that positive attitudes of fieldwork educators can make an essential contribution to an effective and successful fieldwork placement.

Models of student/educator relationships

The most commonly used educational model for fieldwork education is the one-student-to-one-educator relationship. It has traditionally been advocated as the most effective learning model although it seems that there are no clear grounds for this

Table 6.1 Skills and attitudes of fieldwork educators

SKILLS

- competence as a clinician (being a role model)
- organizational skills
- interactional and interpersonal skills (giving feedback which is timely and consistent)
- competence as an educator
- adaptable in approach to the structure of the programme

POSITIVE ATTITUDES	NEGATIVE ATTITUDES
• accessible	• rigid
• enjoys teaching	• stifles originality
• enthusiastic	• controlling
• supportive	• unsupportive
• open	• dominating
• honest	• uncaring
• flexible	• smothering
• empathetic	• restrictive
• accepting	• unconcerned
• sensitive	• insensitive
• patient	• dogmatic
• non-defensive	• arrogant
• committed to their role	• lacking in confidence
• objective	• belittling

Sources: Christie *et al.*, 1985; Kautzmann, 1990; Tarrant, 1990.

assumption. The reason for perpetuating this model seems not to be linked to any perceived educational benefits for the student but to the perception that it is more costly and demanding for the fieldwork educator to have more than one student to manage at a time. Now there is growing awareness that this one-to-one ratio is not necessarily the most effective way of developing a student's knowledge and reasoning skills (Ryan, 1990; 1995) and that a one-to-one ratio is not necessarily the most cost-effective for the service.

One educator to two or more students

Placing two or more students with one fieldwork educator is commonly thought to create double the amount of work for the educator and has been strongly resisted by occupational therapists in the field, although used effectively in other professions such as physiotherapy. However, discussions with fieldwork educators who have used this model have been very positive. Contrary to the belief that this causes more work for the educator, the workload is actually reduced. Each student has both a shared agenda for action and an individual agenda for action, which depends on learning needs and client needs. Students can be set project work to undertake

Table 6.2 Student responses to negative attitudes and experiences

If students were exposed to negative attitudes and experiences they:

- became lazy, 'didn't bother'
- showed reduced enthusiasm for work
- showed reduced motivation/incentive to work
- became withdrawn
- perceived the placement as wasting time
- did not know what was expected
- had no example of how to be an occupational therapist
- felt worthless, unrespected
- had no challenge
- lacked direction
- became too tense to learn
- became disillusioned with the profession
- lost enthusiasm for the course

Table 6.3 Exposure to positive attitudes and meaningful learning

If students were exposed to positive attitudes and meaningful learning experiences on placement they claimed that the experiences:

- increased their self-confidence and their confidence with clients
- helped them gain confidence in their own skills and abilities
- improved their ability to take responsibility
- increased their knowledge and self-awareness
- increased their confidence in making and justifying edcisions
- provided opportunities to make, and learn from mistakes in a safe environment
- developed ideas for them to try in the future
- helped them gain knowledge of their abilities, strengths and points to work on in the future
- helped them gain an understanding of how to be self-directed
- increased their respect for, and positive feelings towards, the profession
- gave them satisfaction in their work
- increased their own professionalism
- increased their understanding of how to become a good fieldwork educator

together and, because they support each other, they can be given more challenging tasks than can often be given to an individual.

The reason for the reduction in demands on the fieldwork educator is that a student's first line of enquiry will almost certainly be to the other student, and not to the fieldwork educator. The students then problem-solve together and re-define their learning needs in the light of their experience. They also support each other personally and professionally during the placement. Although time needs to be made available for individual feedback, much of the feedback and learning can take place in a group. Students tend to learn better from having dialogue, and opportunities for dialogue increase where there is more than one student.

Competition between students is sometimes perceived as a problem but if the situation is managed sensitively it can actually be used to advantage. Increasingly, settings are being sought which are prepared to offer placements to two students simultaneously simply because they support dialogue and provide opportunities for students to learn from each other. This promotes students' professional development without necessarily placing extra strain on the service. This model has been used in Canada for some time (Tiberius and Gaiptman, 1985) and, as Alsop (1994) notes, is also advocated by Harlan and Brinson for the USA.

The group education model

This model provides an opportunity for students to increase knowledge and skills through participating in group learning. It is dynamic and the relationships can be altered according to the needs of both the educators and the students. For most of the day students work with different therapists but come together for group discussions and shared learning. Usually one fieldwork educator facilitates group learning on a daily basis; other groups may be scheduled without a facilitator present. Students coach and support each other and they generate ideas and topics for discussion at subsequent meetings. In this way students' immediate learning needs are addressed.

Group and shared learning has been used in both physical settings (Jung *et al.*, 1994) and mental health settings (Hengel and Romeo, 1995) in Canada and the USA respectively. There are some concerns about the quality of rapport between fieldwork educators and students compared with a 1:1 ratio, and about clarity regarding who takes overall responsibility for a student but these can be overcome. The model has advantages in that it encourages students to take more responsibility for their learning, improves students' confidence and sense of competency and autonomy, and it promotes the development of their individual clinical reasoning skills.

The long-arm model

As its name suggests, this is an educational model which enables students to access fieldwork settings where occupational therapists are not currently working, so the fieldwork educator has to undertake the role from a distance. Given the right circumstances, a structure may be established whereby the student might be guided on a daily basis by a member of another profession, and the Occupational Therapy educator visits regularly to provide professional input and to assist in the assessment of professional competence. This model may be used where students choose to gain experience in non-traditional fieldwork settings. The merits of using such placements and the structures which need to be in place were described in Chapter 4.

Non-occupational therapists as educators

In 1986, Cole Spencer questioned why more use was not being made of other professionals in students' formal education. At a conference she stated:

> our educational process seems to offer little encouragement (and sometimes promotes negative expectations) for learning from members of other disciplines. The tendency may well have negative implications for the later development of good working relationships and teamwork skills by students (p. 108).

The use of non-occupational therapists as role models has tended to be a sensitive issue for the profession. As described in Chapter 4, however, there may be many advantages to students gaining experience in a particular setting where occupational therapists are not currently practising. Students would work alongside a member of another profession on a day-to-day basis and have supervision with an occupational therapist perhaps once a week. The occupational therapist would provide input regarding professional skills and processes and help the student relate their experience specifically to Occupational Therapy practice.

Alsop (1991) reported that students found many advantages in working with non-occupational therapists, for instance they identified that they:

- learned detailed knowledge about various conditions from specialists;
- learned different techniques and approaches used in client care;
- learned different strategies for problem-solving and were able to explore different viewpoints and perspectives to those of the Occupational Therapy profession;
- gained an appreciation of the role of other professionals and insight into the difficulties they experienced;
- learned about the contribution that other professionals made to the multi-disciplinary team.

For these students, working with other professionals was a very positive experience which enabled them to develop knowledge, skills and attitudes relevant to professional practice.

Professional guidelines on models of supervisory relationships

In view of the many changes occurring in fieldwork education the College of Occupational Therapists (1993) made explicit the models of supervisory relationships of which it approved. Three models were advocated: Direct Supervision; Indirect Supervision; and Collaborative Supervision all of which respected the World Federation Standards for Fieldwork Education.

In brief, the Direct Supervision model is where an accredited fieldwork educator is in a direct relationship with a student and takes all responsibility for guiding the student's learning. Indirect Supervision is where an occupational therapist, who may not be accredited, works directly with the student but is supervised in that capacity by an accredited fieldwork educator. In the Collaborative Supervision model an accredited fieldwork educator collaborates with a member of another profession to provide the fieldwork placement. The non-occupational therapist may be a member of the same multi-disciplinary team as the accredited fieldwork educator. The accredited fieldwork educator may alternatively operate in a completely different service to the one in which the student is placed and in which the other professional is based. Long-arm arrangements would then be made. Both the occupational therapist and the other professional would collaborate in teaching and assessing the student. Figure 6.2 shows these relationships in diagrammatic form.

The benefits of having these models are that they make explicit the arrangements

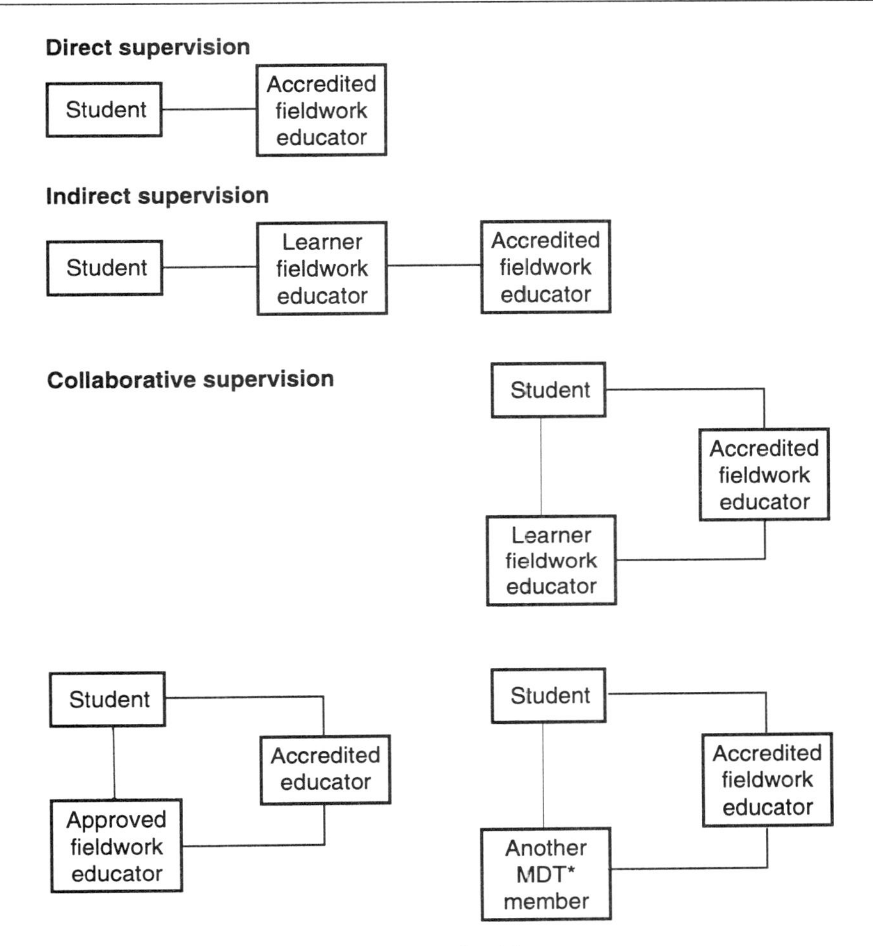

Figure 6.2 Models of supervisor/educator relationships
Reproduced with permission of the College of Occupational Therapists

Source: College of Occupational Therapists, *Guidelines for Assuring the Quality of Fieldwork Education of Occupational Therapy Students,* SSP 165, p. 4.

which the profession permits and they allow a wider range of fieldwork placements to be used without threatening standards of fieldwork education. An alternative, but equally acceptable model, is shown in Figure 6.3. Here, a coordinating fieldwork educator takes overall responsibility for a group of students but involves a number of other educators from the same placement in the students' supervision. The coordinator designs the programme and ensures its implementation, sometimes through a direct relationship with the students and at other times through an indirect relationship as other therapists become involved. Students have access to other students for support as well as having access to a number of fieldwork educators for supervision.

Whatever the arrangement, it is crucial that the profession maintains its standards

Model (a)

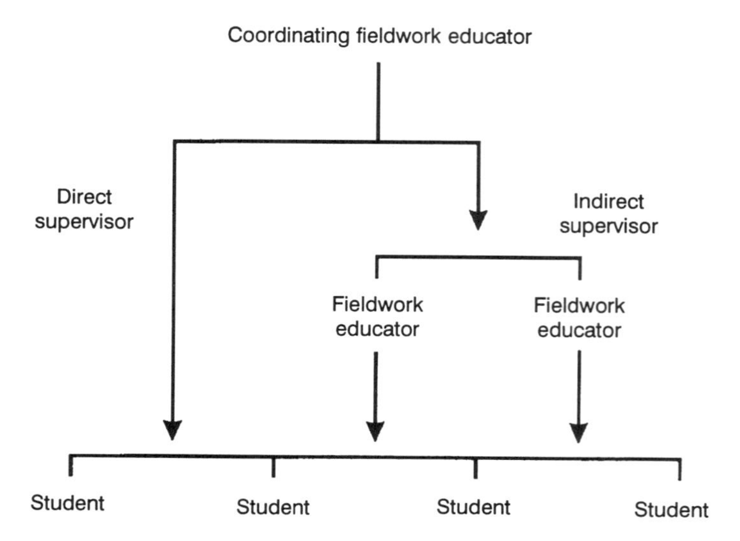

Model (b)

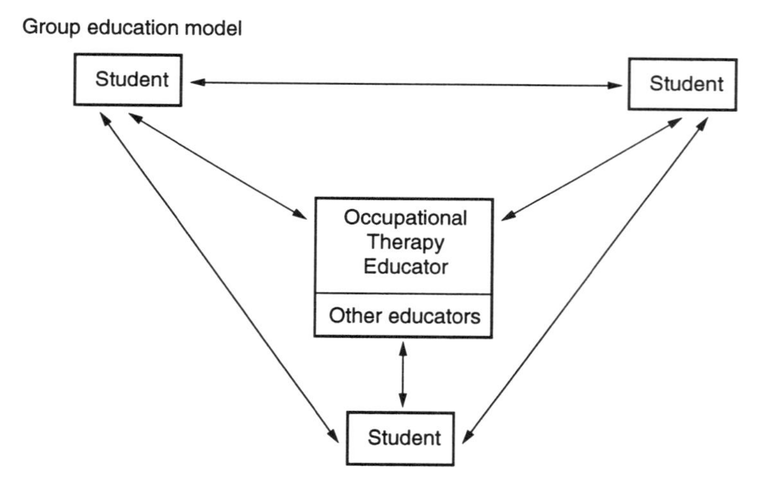

Figure 6.3 Group education models

of practice. Documents specifying standards are available from Professional Bodies. Anyone needing clarification of the standards in a particular country is strongly advised to consult the documentation of the relevant professional organization.

SUMMARY

This chapter has explained how accreditation is a process for assuring quality of fieldwork education and that there is potential for accrediting both the fieldwork placements and fieldwork educators for their role with students. The chapter presented the positive characteristics that are known to be desirable for fieldwork educators to possess and details the functions they are expected to perform. It has been shown that the role of the fieldwork educator extends beyond the role of practitioner and that it is essential for those intending to be involved with student education to develop their knowledge, particularly of adult learning theories, and skills. Many different student/educator models are possible. The models approved by the profession have been outlined and other possible models, such as group and long-arm models of student education, have been described.

REFERENCES

Alsop, A. (1991) *Five Schools Project: Clinical Practice Curriculum Development.* Unpublished report, Dorset House School of Occupational Therapy, Oxford.

Alsop, A. (1994) The Fieldwork Experience CAN-AM Conference 1994: cultural connections. *British Journal of Occupational Therapy*, **57**(8), 320.

Burnard, P. (1994) *Counselling Skills for Health Professionals*, 2nd edn. Chapman & Hall, London.

Christiansen, C. and Christiansen P. (1994) Canada: the OT's perspective. *OT Week*, **8**(26), 20–3.

Christie, B. A., Joyce, P. C. and Moeller, P. L (1985) Fieldwork experience part 11: the supervisors' dilemma. *American Journal of Occupational Therapy*, **39**(10), 675–81.

Cole Spencer, J. (1986) Perceptions of a recent graduate: a broad activity analysis of occupational therapy education. In *Target 2000 – Promoting Excellence in Education.* Proceedings, 22–6 June, American Occupational Therapy Association, Rockville MD.

College of Occupational Therapists (1991) *Statement on the Management of Occupational Therapy Services and on Fieldwork Education.* SPP, 161, College of Occupational Therapists, London.

College of Occupational Therapists (1993) *Guidelines for Assuring the Quality of the Fieldwork Education of Occupational Therapy Students.* SPP, 165, College of Occupational Therapists, London.

College of Occupational Therapists (1994) *Recommended Requirements for the Accreditation of Fieldwork Educators.* SPP, 166, College of Occupational Therapists, London.

College of Occupational Therapists (1995) *Code of Ethics and Professional Conduct for Occupational Therapists.* College of Occupational Therapists, London.

Edwards, M. and Baptiste, S. (1987) The occupational therapist as a clinical teacher. *Canadian Journal of Occupational Therapy*, **54**(5), 249–55.

Frum, D. C. and Opacich, K. J. (1987) *Supervision: Development of Therapeutic Competence*. The American Occupational Therapy Association Inc., Baltimore, USA.

Graves, S (1994) Accreditation goes independent. *OT Week*, **8**(18), 20-Ô1.

Hengel, J. L. and Romeo, J. L. (1995) A group approach to mental health fieldwork. *American Journal of Occupational Therapy*, **49**(4), 354–8.

Ilott, I. (1995) Fail or not to fail? A course for fieldwork educators. *American Journal of Occupational Therapy*, **49**(3), 250–5.

Jung, B., Martin, A., Graden., L. and Awrey, J. (1994) Fieldwork Education: a shared supervision model. *Canadian Journal of Occupational Therapy*, **61**(1), 12–19.

Kautzmann, L. N. (1990) Clinical teaching: fieldwork supervisors' attitudes and values. *American Journal of Occupational Therapy*, **44**(9), 835–8.

Ryan, S. (1990) *Clinical Reasoning: A Descriptive Study Comparing Novice and Experienced Occupational Therapists*. Unpublished master's thesis, Columbia University, USA.

Ryan, S. (1995) Teaching clinical reasoning to occupational therapists during fieldwork education. In Higgs, J. and Jones. M. (1995) *Clinical Reasoning in the Health Professions*. Butterworth-Heinemann, Oxford.

Tiberius, R. and Gaiptman, B. (1985) The supervisor-student ratio 1:1 versus 1:2. *Canadian Journal of Occupational Therapy*, **52**, 179–83.

Wallis, M. (1987) 'Profession' and 'Professionalism' and the emerging profession of occupational therapy: Part 1. *British Journal of Occupational Therapy*, **50**(8), 254–5.

PART TWO

The Fieldwork Experience

Setting the scene: expectations of you and others

7

This chapter covers:

- the placement as a context for both learning and service delivery;
- expectations of the placement and the fieldwork educator;
- expectations of the university;
- your responsibilities in preparing for the placement;
- clients' rights and needs.

As with many things in life, the more thorough the preparation for an event, the more likely it is to be successful. But in order for you to be able to prepare for an event such as fieldwork you need to be informed about what you might expect. The purpose of this chapter is therefore to set the scene for your fieldwork placement and provide you with relevant information about factors which might influence your overall experience.

It is one thing to think about your placement as an extension of the educational environment where learning needs can be met, it is quite another to see the placement as a working environment which has a primary aim of delivering services to clients. Yet they are one and the same thing. We must therefore encourage you to view the placement in the context of service delivery and to appreciate how both clients' needs and your needs have to be managed at the same time. You will then appreciate the expectations that people have of you and the kind of preparations you need to make for the placement to be a success.

EXPECTATIONS OF YOUR PLACEMENT

Before we discuss the expectations and responsibilities of the different people involved in your fieldwork education, just stop for a moment and consider what you are really expecting of your fieldwork placement and fieldwork educator, and what others may expect of you.

Perhaps in thinking through your expectations you noted that you would want your fieldwork placement to be well organized and to be one which will provide you with a variety of good learning experiences. You might also have noted that you would expect your fieldwork educator to be properly qualified, to be experienced, to act as a role model for you, to be supportive and to be in a position to guide you as you learn to work with clients. Almost certainly you would expect your fieldwork educator to take a particular interest in you as a person, and in your progress, and to make time in his or her busy schedule to give you constructive feedback on your performance. This is the time in your educational programme when you can practise your skills under supervision of an experienced practitioner in the relative safety of a supportive environment. You probably feel that your fieldwork experience is an important part of your education and that all efforts in the placement should be directed towards ensuring that it meets your specific learning needs. But as we have explained there are many other factors which have to be taken into consideration.

Balancing service and student needs

Everyone will aim to ensure that your fieldwork experience is of high quality, but you need to keep in mind that service delivery to clients takes precedence over everything. High workload levels are often quoted both informally and formally by occupational therapists as one of the main influences on a decision not to supervise students. The reality is that you can expect your fieldwork educator to have a considerable caseload of clients as well as taking responsibility for your fieldwork education. Fieldwork educators must therefore balance and prioritize the needs and demands made of them in the service and keep all their various responsibilities in perspective. Your needs as a student will be addressed in relation to everything else, but not always as a matter of priority.

Idealistic and realistic expectations

University staff are very aware of the problems faced by occupational therapists engaged in service delivery, and the various demands made on their time. Expectations made of them by academic staff and students therefore have to be realistic. This can sometimes mean that placements may seem to fall short of an ideal if expectations are high, but this does not necessarily mean that the learning experience for the student will in any way be inadequate.

Sometimes students' expectations of placements can be rather idealistic. For instance, students can make what can seem to be unreasonable demands of a fieldwork educator in terms of time for teaching and supervision. Students sometimes expect to be taught theoretical knowledge by the fieldwork educator rather than to search it out in the literature for themselves. The fieldwork educator will almost certainly expect you to take responsibility for that kind of learning. Students can also be demanding of the educator's attention for answering questions, providing explanations and for giving feedback. Perceptions of adequate levels of attention and supervision vary. This is why it is essential for you to reach some agreement with your fieldwork educator about the timing of discussions and the nature of supervision early in the placement. Ideally it should be written into the placement contract.

We want you to note that there can actually be advantages to students having what they might consider to be a 'less than ideal' placement, depending on the circumstances. For instance, where everything runs smoothly in a service you could easily be lulled into a false sense of security about what life in a busy organization is really like. If, on the other hand, you are exposed to the dilemmas of service provision, the demands on staff time, and the reality of work pressures at an early stage in your career you will be better prepared for such a life when qualified. There is no point in protecting yourself from the hard realities of life in employment while you are a student. You need to learn to cope as much with service pressures and demands as with delivering client care while you are on placement.

THE UNIVERSITY'S EXPECTATIONS OF FIELDWORK EDUCATORS AND PLACEMENTS

Given that the service offering the placement has a primary duty to clients there are still some basic requirements that should be met in the placement for it to become a learning environment for you and a suitable setting for your fieldwork education. The university therefore expects:

- that a named occupational therapist will take responsibility for your supervision;
- that the fieldwork educator has the relevant experience and is willing to accept you as a student and fulfil the responsibilities of the educator role;
- that the staff in the service operate to an Equal Opportunities Policy;
- that the service maintains good standards of practice and operates a policy for staff development;
- that the service is able to provide you with relevant experience which meets the objectives of the placement;
- that the fieldwork educator communicates adequately with university staff and seeks to understand the programme of study which you are following and the assessment procedures involved;
- that the fieldwork educator manages and facilitates your learning, takes time to give you regular feedback on your performance and evaluates your practice fairly and as objectively as possible.

These are usually considered to be the minimum expectations for a placement but as we have mentioned already, some universities operate a more stringent accreditation system where extra criteria have to be met by services which provide placements.

Benefits and costs of student education

The provision of fieldwork placements is generally perceived by service managers to incur **costs** in terms of staff time and training expenses, while the **benefits** of receiving students into the service remain unacknowledged. A study carried out in 1993 by Walker and Cooper concluded that, on balance, there were gains for services which provided fieldwork education for Occupational Therapy students, although service managers do not necessarily accept this conclusion. Since managers tend only to see the costs involved in providing student placements it is not uncommon for charges to be made for fieldwork education. However, there are centres which believe that providing student education enhances the quality of the service provided to clients and helps with the recruitment of staff to the department. Where this is so, fieldwork education is recognized as acceptable staff activity and fieldwork educators are supported in their role.

EXPECTATIONS OF THE UNIVERSITY

Fieldwork educators like to be well prepared for receiving students so they welcome early contact with the university about the placement. Good communication helps the fieldwork educator to plan a programme which accords with learning objectives established for the placement and ensures that specific needs of the student can be integrated into the programme at the planning stage. In order to carry out their role effectively, fieldwork educators have certain expectations of the university. They expect university staff:

- to be well organized with their arrangements for fieldwork education;
- to maintain close links with services and service staff;
- to provide relevant and timely information about placements;
- to provide education and training for prospective fieldwork educators;
- to support educators and students during the fieldwork placement;
- to respond promptly to problems being experienced by a student on placement;
- to keep them informed of curriculum developments;
- to keep up-to-date with current issues relating to practice and service provision.

Competition for placements can be fierce. This means that services may choose to work only with universities which are well organized and efficient in the way they manage fieldwork education.

EXPECTATIONS OF YOU AS A STUDENT

Having discussed some of the expectations of other people involved with fieldwork, now it is time to examine what other people expect of you. Once you know the expectations you should be able to prepare to meet them. At the beginning of the chapter we asked you to think about these expectations. The following are some of the points which you might have thought of. There are expectations:

- that you come well-prepared for the placement, having read up about the conditions you might expect to see;
- that you behave and dress according to the conventions of the service;
- that you engage in the placement and take advantage of the learning opportunities it offers;
- that you demonstrate a commitment to learning and professional development;

- that you take responsibility for your learning, engaging in reflection and honest self-evaluation of your performance and behaviour;
- that you are able to accept constructive criticism and are prepared to modify behaviour as a result;
- that you are punctual for appointments, and keep other people informed in the event of difficulties;
- that you integrate into the service team and respect the needs of its members;
- that you take responsibility according to your stage of training, but acknowledge the limits of your responsibility and experience so as not to endanger yourself or other people;
- that you work in accordance with the Code of Ethics and Professional Conduct;
- that you are inquisitive, and demonstrate an enquiring mind, and that you are prepared to develop your repertoire of skills and knowledge using the resources around you.

These are just some of the expectations of you. Overall, there are expectations that you will present and act as a professional person, and develop knowledge, skills and attitudes in an appropriate way.

TAKING RESPONSIBILITY FOR YOURSELF AND YOUR LEARNING

You will realize by now that fieldwork education is an integral part of the total curriculum for the course and that you are expected to approach fieldwork with the same commitment as for the academic programme, if not more. This means participating actively in your fieldwork studies, and taking responsibility for your learning.

As a student on placement you are a representative of your Occupational Therapy course and of the educational establishment in which it is based. You are expected to perform as a responsible, reliable, professional person who respects the clients, staff and the service with which you are placed. You have a responsibility, therefore, to act as an ambassador for your university, acknowledging and adhering to the standards that it sets for its students. Your cooperation and responsible attitude are not only qualities to be promoted for your own benefit and your own professional development, they are also qualities which will help ensure that good working relationships are maintained between fieldwork and academic staff for the benefit of future students.

PREPARING FOR THE PLACEMENT

It would be quite natural for you to experience feelings of anxiety as you anticipate your first, and even a subsequent, fieldwork placement. A range of emotions is commonly experienced by students prior to fieldwork. If you talk to your colleagues you can expect them to feel the same way as you. We say more about how you can deal with feelings of anxiety in Chapter 8. However, the emotions you feel about fieldwork education might also include excitement about the prospect of using newfound knowledge in the workplace and of practising new skills alongside colleagues. Through your work with clients you have the opportunity to develop both personally and professionally. Preparing adequately for the placement, engaging actively in fieldwork and communicating openly with your fieldwork educator should help you settle into the placement.

COPING WITH THE UNEXPECTED

The reality of work life in a busy service can mean that you might find yourself having to cope with unexpected difficulties. Students have reported (Alsop, 1991) that sorting themselves out when they were in difficult or demanding situations taught them a good deal about themselves and their ability to cope. Their self-confidence increased and the experience taught them how to use effective negotiating and coping strategies to see them through the situation. Mitchell and Kampfe (1990, 1993) found that Occupational Therapy students frequently employed effective problem-focused coping strategies in an effort to control their environment. As a student you may well find yourself in a predicament during your placement, taking a decision on your own or taking action unexpectedly. This can lead you into a process of self-discovery where you gain new insights into your own ability to cope. If this should happen to you, treat it as a positive learning experience.

THE NEEDS AND RIGHTS OF CLIENTS

Everyone concerned with fieldwork education (yourself, academic staff, service managers, fieldwork educators, sponsors of education and training, and sometimes employers) has expectations about the delivery of fieldwork education. These must be acknowledged. You will also be involved with clients and they, too, have needs, rights and expectations.

Meeting the needs of clients in the most efficient and effective way is a prime concern of health and social care staff. You will almost certainly find that health care staff with whom you are placed work under enormous pressures to cope with high levels of referrals, long waiting lists and other demands on their time. Whatever the demands the care and service given to clients must be of a consistently good standard, and must not in any way fall below safe levels. Whoever is responsible for care provision must be competent to provide that care to a safe standard, and that includes students.

This is why it is important for you to check exactly what is expected of you during fieldwork. You must clarify concerns, and discuss with your fieldwork educator any limitations which you think you have which may affect the quality and standard of care provided to clients. The fieldwork educator has a duty not to put clients at risk and must ensure that any instruction given to you as a student can be carried out safely and effectively. The fieldwork educator is still the therapist responsible for client care so must delegate appropriately.

Clients have a right afforded to them by the Patient's Charter (1991) to decline to be treated by medical students. This right can be extended to include Occupational Therapy students so it is essential for you to clarify the extent of your role within the service and the way in which you should introduce yourself to clients. You have a responsibility to work professionally, safely and to an acceptable standard of competence despite your student status. If you have any doubts about this then you must discuss your concerns with your fieldwork educator who has overall responsibility for clients in his or her care.

SUPPORT FOR FIELDWORK EDUCATORS

Fieldwork education is provided as a partnership between fieldwork educators, the university and the student. All have expectations of others and all have responsibilities themselves which they must take. Fieldwork educators usually enjoy their involvement with students (Alsop, 1991) and, despite the problems which inevitably arise, often find supervising students to be a positive experience. The extended role and associated responsibilities provide practitioners with opportunities for professional development and for widening their experience of professional practice. In order to do their job well, however, they need, and should expect to be supported by their service manager and by academic staff in the important role which they play in the process of student education.

SUMMARY

This chapter has explained that fieldwork education takes place in the context of a service provided to clients. Students' needs take second place to client care which must continue to be delivered to a safe and acceptable standard despite student involvement. All those who play a part in fieldwork education have their own responsibilities. They also have expectations of others in the role that they fulfil. As a result, fieldwork education becomes a partnership between the university, the service offering the placement and the student. Given an understanding of these expectations and responsibilities, students should appreciate how to prepare themselves for the placement so that they can take advantage of the learning opportunities it offers.

REFERENCES

Alsop, A. (1991) *The Five Schools Project: Clinical Practice Curriculum Development.* Unpublished report, Dorset House School of Occupational Therapy, Oxford.

Mitchell, M. and Kampfe, C. (1990) Coping strategies used by occupational therapy students during fieldwork: an exploratory study. *American Journal of Occupational Therapy*, **44**(6), 543–50.

Mitchell, M. and Kampfe, C. (1993) Student coping strategies and perceptions of fieldwork. *American Journal of Occupational Therapy*, **47**(6), 535-40.

The Patients Charter (1991) Department of Health, HMSO, London.

Walker, C. and Cooper, F. (1993) Fieldwork education: to charge or not to charge? *British Journal of Occupational Therapy*, **56**(2), 51–4.

8 Examining your needs

This chapter covers:

- an overview of personal needs during fieldwork;
- an examination of intra-personal, inter-personal, psychological and physical health needs while on placement;
- strategies to maintain good health.

This chapter deals with more personal aspects of the fieldwork experience. We give you ideas about how to discover and examine your intra-personal and interpersonal needs, and your psychological and physical reactions to them so that you can begin to understand them better. This knowledge should help you to become more aware of yourself and your needs before, during and after a placement, and ultimately to see how you might use this understanding of yourself within the therapeutic relationship. As you probably know, one of the central tenets of the Occupational Therapy profession is that, as a therapist, you should consider the **whole** person when you are working with your clients. In this chapter we want you to consider the **whole** of you so that, as you become aware of your different needs, you will start to feel more in control of the fieldwork situation. We have included some interactional exercises in this chapter to help you to gain some understanding of these different needs.

The chapter is fairly long so it is divided into five sections as follows:

Section 1 provides an overview of personal needs;
Section 2 examines your intra-personal needs;
Section 3 explores your inter-personal needs;
Section 4 addresses your psychological needs;
Section 5 relates to your physical health needs.

Giving consideration to all these needs together should help you to gain some real understanding of yourself as you prepare for the fieldwork experience. Figure 8.1 provides an overview of the different needs.

Intrapersonal needs	**Interpersonal needs**
• Values, beliefs – attitudes, behaviours	• Relationship with educator
• Reasons for entering the profession	• Support: peer, mentor
• Personal theories about practice	**Psychological needs**
• Need to be valued and accepted	• Managing anxiety
• Need for success	• Controlling tiredness
Physical health needs	• Being quiet, calm
• Vaccinations	• Family contact
• Universal precautions against HIV / AIDS	• Personal problems
• Health preservation	• Managing stress
• Back care	• Avoiding burnout

Figure 8.1 An overview of personal needs

1. OVERVIEW OF YOUR PERSONAL NEEDS

The examination of students' personal needs from their own perspective is one of the most neglected areas of study. Only a few articles, and even fewer research projects, have been written on this topic in the Occupational Therapy literature. We want to highlight its importance, but before we introduce some exercises that will help you to become more aware of yourself, we would like to mention some of the published work on the subject, and the survey that we undertook before we started this book.

From the few studies that have been written, one described how **anticipated** anxiety often develops before fieldwork starts (Greenstein, 1983). Another (Muldary, 1983) identified inter-personal conflicts as being a significant source of stress that leads to **burnout**. A further study in physiotherapy described student burnout and noted how it could be spotted and managed (Brust, 1986). In 1990, Yuen suggested that students could be better equipped for coping with fieldwork through the use of seminars about different aspects of burnout held at university before the start of a placement. In view of these findings, we have included sections about anxiety, stress and burnout in this chapter. You can see that some published work has already addressed reasons for students' anxieties. Before we started this book we wanted to be clear about what some of those anxieties might be so that we, too, could address them in some way. We therefore consulted students about their personal concerns before they went on their fieldwork placement. Here is a summary of what they said. They were concerned about:

- whether the expectations of the supervisors would be too high for their level of knowledge;
- whether there would be emotional support;
- what the expectations of supervision would be;
- where they would be working;
- what they would be doing;
- what their level of independence would be;
- whether they would be expected to carry a caseload and how big it would be;
- what the role of the therapist was in the department;
- what their role would be;
- what would happen if there was a personality clash;
- what would happen if they got lost in paperwork;
- what they would do if there was insufficient guidance – or too much guidance;
- how they should interact with clients;
- what they would do if they didn't know enough;
- whether they would get on with the team;
- what they would do if things went wrong;
- what they would do if the supervisor was a 'dragon';
- whether there were guidelines for the assessment;
- whether there would be any other students at the same placement.

You may identify personally with some of these concerns. They seem to be quite common and substantiate Greenstein's (1983) study that anxiety often develops before the start of fieldwork. There is clearly a 'need' for information and for coping strategies which, as Yuen (1990) proposes, could be addressed in a briefing session before the placement starts. Being aware of your concerns, and knowing that others anticipate fieldwork in much the same way as you, should help you manage your anxieties. You should also remember that both your fieldwork coordinator and your fieldwork educator will understand these anxieties too.

Having made a note of concerns commonly expressed by students, we can now return to focus on you. The next section will help you to get to know more about yourself in a different way as part of the overview of your personal needs. Later in the chapter we return to the issue of anxiety and how to deal with it.

Getting to know yourself

Getting to know yourself and being in touch with your own needs has another purpose. It is an important part of your development as a health professional. The more you know about, and understand yourself, the better you will be as a therapist. The phrase 'the professional use of self' is often referred to as an important aspect of therapy (Schwartzberg, 1992) and as such, has a place in both qualifying and continuing professional education programmes. One way of becoming more aware of yourself and seeing yourself as others see you is by using the Johari Window designed by Joseph Luft (1969) which is shown in Figure 8.2. It focuses attention on both your private self and your public self.

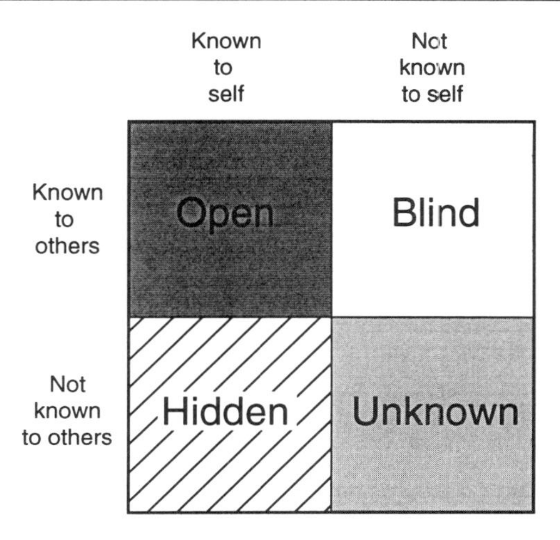

Figure 8.2 The Johari Window
Reprinted/adapted by permission

Source: from Barker, L. (1987) *Communication,* 4th edn. Allyn and Bacon

The OPEN section represents aspects of yourself that you know about and that you are willing to share with others. The HIDDEN section represents other aspects of yourself which you know about but which you are not willing to share with others. The BLIND section represents information about yourself of which you are unaware but which others know about you. The UNKNOWN section represents what is unknown to both yourself and others.

Exercise: Finding out about yourself
Draw out two windows for yourself and ask someone else to fill in the BLIND section on one of them and in it describe how they see you, your strengths and weaknesses, what they like about you and what is annoying. You can keep this exercise fairly general if you like, or you can ask them to provide specific information, for example, about how you appear at team meetings. While they are doing this, fill in the OPEN and HIDDEN sections yourself, writing down how you think you appear to others. Then in private examine both windows. Check in the BLIND section for statements that you had not written in the other two sections. This exercise will really illustrate any assets or shortcomings that you need to be aware of. The more you do become aware of how others see you, the more you will be able to change the shape of your BLIND and UNKNOWN windows.

This exercise should help you to be more aware of your interactions with your peers and colleagues in certain situations. It should also increase your ability to be **empathetic** with the clients you work with, so that you become more involved in their present life story. You can repeat this exercise each time you go on placement because you will develop personally and professionally over time and your perceptions will change. Now that we have given an overview, let us take a closer look at your inner needs which we will refer to as your intra-personal needs

2. INTRA-PERSONAL NEEDS: YOUR VALUES AND BELIEFS

Intra-personal needs are those that are inside you; needs that you often do not or cannot acknowledge, and yet they are there. These needs are more important than they might first appear. They reflect your physical, emotional, cognitive and social needs, in fact they form your personality (Barker, 1987).

Throughout your life you have been developing values and beliefs which are important to you. They have been shaped by your personal life experiences, 'your personal framework' (Popper, as cited in Young and Quinn, 1992) and by exposure to other points of view. These values are deeply embedded and often manifest themselves as behavioural attitudes towards people and objects. Values are often very hard to recognize in yourself. Sometimes it takes other people to point them out to you. Undesirable or negative beliefs can be hard to change, but what you can change is the way you show them in your behaviour. It is important to realize this as you meet people in the fieldwork setting.

If you answer the questions in the following exercise you will build up another picture of yourself.

Exercise: Your beliefs

Write down your immediate responses to the questions and statements below:

About people

Q1 Do you like people and feel comfortable with them, especially people you don't know?

Q2 Can you think of any group of people you do not feel at ease with?

About health

Q3 What do you believe makes people healthy?

Q4 What are the major components of health?

Q5 Do these components apply to you and do you think you are healthy?

About therapy

Q6 What do you think are the major goals of therapy?

Q7 Describe any therapy you have seen that illustrates your response to question 6.

About recovery

Q8 List the major factors that influence recovery.

Q9 From the list above separate the factors that are:
intrinsic (coming from within the person) or
extrinsic (coming from an outside source)

About care

Q10 How much do you think a caring attitude helps a client in **their** recovery?

Q11 Can you think of any instances when caring would not help?

Do this exercise alone and then share your responses with a partner. Think about any differences in your answers and discuss the reasons for these. You may have absorbed some of these values without even realizing. As your professional education develops it will be interesting for you to see if your values change.

Attitudes

Your values are reflected in your attitudes and they manifest themselves in your behaviour. Sometimes on a fieldwork placement you may be confronted with situations that you would normally choose to avoid, or you might have to work with a group of people that you have no previous experience of interacting with at all. Although you may be unaware of them you might have some very stereotypical ideas or biases that you have acquired from various sources such as relatives, friends, characters on television or in films, people you have noticed, lived or worked with.

Exercise: your attitudes
Think about the following groups of people, write down what you **feel** about them.

- Babies and young children.
- Elderly people.
- Sick people.
- Poor people.
- People from other cultures.
- People with different religions.

Have you written down things or even thought of things that should go into your hidden Johari Window?

The purpose of these exercises is for you to imagine how you might react as a student if you work with clients who have some of the attributes that you feel negative about. You will need to examine your negative or neutral feelings about people. They often come from a lack of understanding or from an inadequate knowledge base. You can do something about them by becoming better informed. Try to find out who to talk to, places you might visit or books or articles you might read.

Before we continue, take a moment to look at the things that you and others have listed under your strengths in your Johari Window. Some of these may surprise you, others you may feel relatively comfortable about. Being aware of, and using these strengths during your fieldwork placement will give you added confidence. Let us go on and consider other aspects of your self knowledge which relate to fieldwork.

Choice of profession

Everyone has a different reason for entering the profession, but this is something you may not have thought very much about since making that decision. It is also an area not well researched. Some of your answers in the previous exercises may give you clues to your personal reason for wishing to become an occupational therapist. Understanding the reason behind your decision will help you identify and deal with **mismatches** as they occur on placement. A mismatch occurs when two people come to the same situation with different expectations which do not match. It manifests itself, for instance, when a client with whom you are working will not cooperate with the therapy session you have planned. The likely explanation is that each of you wants something different, but you are not aware of it. In the next sections we highlight some of the reasons why mismatches occur and explain how important it is for you to understand what is happening.

The altruistic mismatch

For some students many of their values are coloured by altruistic feelings of 'doing good to others'. If left unexamined, these feelings can paint a very unreal picture of real situations. When confronted with a situation where the **actual image** of the person you are working with does not fit your **ideal image** a mismatch of values and expectations occurs on both sides. This is when you, or even a qualified therapist, might get 'stuck' and not know how to proceed because the client appears to be uncooperative. Unwittingly, you may be putting your own needs or values onto the needs of the other person. This is why you should be able to recognize and deal with your own needs appropriately.

The 'doing to' and 'doing with' mismatch

Another aspect of practice that can be compromised by your values is the relationship between you and your client. You will see in the professional literature many references to **client-centred** care. This mode of working means that you and the client are addressing problems together, hence the expression 'doing with' (Mattingly, 1994). This way of working emphasizes **collaborative practice** as opposed to **prescriptive practice**. Prescriptive practice is where the therapist decides what the problems are and then works on them but with little consultation with the client.

The professional mismatch

Even if you have not yet been on a fieldwork placement you may have formed some sort of personal framework about the way in which practice should proceed. This may have come from your life experience, from your lecturers, from peers, or from a visit to a placement. As you progress in your professional education, consciously or unconsciously, you will subtly change in the way you think, and sometimes in the way you feel, dress, and behave. We would like you to examine this framework. Problems have arisen on placement because the student's personal idea of practice has not fitted with the way the fieldwork educator likes to work. This is another form of mismatch to which Schon (1987) refers. He suggests that, in some professions, awareness of uncertainty, complexity, instability, uniqueness, and value conflict has led to the emergence of professional pluralism. Competing views of professional practice – competing images of the professional role, the central values of the profession, the relevant knowledge and skills – have come into good currency.

This excerpt illustrates the fact that not all professionals have the same view of practice. The therapist's ideas may be different from your own or from those described at university. It is important that you are aware that this mismatch can happen, and equally important that you do not ignore any conflicting thoughts or feelings. If you do, they may simmer away and affect your performance and ultimately the way that you are seen by others. You would be wise to note any differences in perception and raise them in supervision, or when you are visited by a university tutor. You can then set your perceptions against those of others. Discussing them with others will also help you to put things into perspective and form some judgements about what needs to be done.

Differences and difficulties stand out in the fieldwork setting more than anywhere else. It is one thing to be exposed to new or differing ideas in a university because there is time for debate. It is entirely different when you are on placement and you have to act quickly. You will have to adjust from being a student at university to being a student on placement. Table 8.1 highlights some of the differences noted by Cohn (1993). For instance, you will have to cope with different people and different ways of doing things. You will even be perceived differently, not as a student but as a developing professional.

Professional growth

Professional growth encompasses a range of features such as the development of:

- professional attitudes and behaviour;
- professional confidence and competence;
- the ability to manage learning effectively;
- the motivation to seek knowledge and to develop and improve professional expertise;
- the ability to take initiative;
- skills of inquiry, analysis and problem-solving;
- independence of thought and action, and an ability to be self-reliant;
- the ability to request and use professional support appropriately;
- the ability to operate in accordance with professional standards and code of ethics;
- the ability to evaluate your own professional skills, behaviour and performance;
- the ability to relate to others with sensitivity and respect;

Table 8.1 Distinctions between academic and clinical settings

	Academic setting	*Clinical setting*
Purpose	Facilitate dissemination of knowledge, development of creative thought and student growth, award degrees	Provide high-quality patient care
Faculty/supervisor accountability	1. To student 2. To university	1. To patient and families 2. To clinical center 3. To student
Student accountability	To self	To patients and families, supervisor and clinical center
Pace	Dependent on curriculum; adaptable to student and faculty needs	Dependent on patient needs; less adaptable
Student/educator ratio	Many students to one faculty member	One student to one supervisor
Source of feedback	Summative at midterm or at the end of term; provided by faculty	Provided by patients and families, supervisor, and other staff; formative
Degree of faculty/ supervisor control of educational experience	Able to plan, controlled	Limited control; various diagnoses and lengths of patient stay
Primary learning tools	Books, lectures, audiovisual aids, case studies, simulation	Situation of practice; patients, families and staff
Conceptual learning	Abstract, theoretical	Pragmatic, applied in interpersonal context
Learning process	Teacher-directed	Patient-, self-, and supervisor-directed
Tolerance for ambiguity/uncertainty	High	Low
Lifestyle	Flexible to plan time around class schedule	Structured; flexible time limited to evenings and weekends

Reprinted with permission from Lippincott-Raven Publishers, Philadelphia.
Source: from Cohn, E. (1993) Distinctions between academic and clinical settings. In *Willard and Spackman's Occupational Therapy*, 8th edn, 1993.

- personal clinical reasoning skills;
- the ability to integrate knowledge of theory and practice, and to transfer knowledge and skills from one situation to another;
- depth and breadth of professional knowledge and understanding.

Many fieldwork assessment (evaluation) forms have sections about professional development or professional growth. Look carefully at your own form to see what is expected of you in this area. In the United States one third of the evaluation form focuses on attitude, i.e. the degree to which the student exhibits professional behaviors and attitudes during the performance of the task (AOTA, 1987). It is also highlighted by the results of a research study (Ilott, 1988) which examined the criteria for failing a student on placement. Behaviour problems were listed as the single most frequent reason. You can see, therefore, that **how** you perform a task is at least as important as the outcome of the task. Through your professional growth you will be expected to develop and demonstrate the attitudes and behaviours of an occupational therapist.

Being valued professionally

Another need is that of being accepted and being valued as a contributing member of the professional team. If you return to your Johari Window and review the things you have written in the HIDDEN window you may get a sense of how much you need to be valued, accepted and liked. When you are on your fieldwork placement you will receive formal feedback from your fieldwork educator about your personal performance, but you will also pick up informal and often unspoken signs from others, such as doctors or clients.

You will recognize these signs from the tone of their voice, the frequency of their interaction with you and from how consistently you gain eye contact with them. However, you should be aware that when you are unfamiliar with a situation, and the people in it, you might attribute some of these attitudes to yourself because of your need to be accepted. Other people's reactions might have nothing to do with you at all. Try to stand back from the situation and see if the same person is behaving with others as he or she does towards you. This will help you to put things into perspective. If you think that reactions are triggered by your presence you might consult your BLIND window to see what other people have written about you. Discuss your perceptions with a friend or your fieldwork educator. Always be specific, do not generalize. Use examples such as:

> Did you see Mrs******'s reaction to my suggestion about the activity I planned this morning, is there any way I could have done or said that differently?

You will find this way of getting feedback to be much more straightforward. It will then be up to you to act on the information you receive.

Your need for success

How important is it to you to be successful? You might have written something about this in your HIDDEN window. Everybody has different values about success, and success can be perceived in many different ways. Success is usually interpreted as doing well on placement. Schwartz (1984) believes that you have to work hard to succeed, it doesn't come naturally. On fieldwork placement it is often how well you have prepared yourself, and not just in the academic sense, that makes all the difference.

One of the ways of measuring success is by looking at how much you have learned during the placement. It is important to realize that successful learning can also occur on placements which you consider to be poor; the learning may be successful when the experience was not (Boud *et al.*, 1985; Weimer, 1994).

3. INTER-PERSONAL NEEDS

Most people who choose to work in the health professions or in social care enjoy the company of other people. Sometimes in the literature you see these professions referred to as 'people professions'. Most of us need the stimulation of others' company. Most of our life is spent living directly with others – our family, our peers, our colleagues. The rest of our interactional time is spent indirectly within the society in which we live and work. On fieldwork placement you will spend time with clients and your fieldwork educator so this part of the chapter looks at the inter-personal needs that might arise in this context.

The supervisory relationship

The supervisory relationship, that is the relationship between you and your fieldwork educator, is at the core of the fieldwork experience and is of critical importance (Frum and Opacich, 1987). Loganbill *et al.* (1982) describe it as an intensive, interpersonally focused, one-to-one relationship in which one person is designated to facilitate the development of therapeutic competence in the other person.

In a study by Wallis and Hutchings (1990) students ranked this relationship as the single most important factor that helped them come to terms with the reality of practice. Most of the time you will not be able to choose your fieldwork educator. You will be in this important relationship with less control than you would normally have in other relationships. Within the relationship it is important that your fieldwork educator views you as a person and values you as a distinct individual, rather than categorizing you as 'just another student'. There are things you can do to help this relationship to develop. For instance, you can send your fieldwork educator a concise profile of yourself before you arrive for the placement, so that he or she can begin to relate to you as a person.

Your need for support

We have already highlighted instances where, during fieldwork, you might feel particularly vulnerable. Most of the time, however, you will feel less vulnerable if you have support. We have outlined below some arrangements that you can make for yourself before you go on placement to help you gain this support.

Choosing a mentor

The term **mentor** comes from Greek mythology when Odysseus entrusted his friend, Mentor, with the education of his son Telemachus. A mentor is thus a very special person in a very special relationship with another, someone dedicated to the personal and professional growth of the other (Javernick, 1994). A mentor is sought out for being able to develop the protégé's knowledge, skills and aspirations. He or she is also trustworthy and able to act as a source of comfort to the person mentored (Robertson, 1994). The person chosen to mentor another is often, but need not be, from the same profession. It should, however, be someone who is accessible and committed to that special relationship.

A mentor would be someone you could call on for support or to help you see your way through problems. That person should be someone you admire, possibly someone you aspire to be like. The person may be from your university, from a previous placement or from a place of work. He or she does not have to be familiar with your programme or your placement but should have had sufficient work experience to understand your needs and give suggestions for resolving problems which might arise. Normally you would ask this person formally if he or she would be a mentor to you and act as a source of guidance and support.

Arranging a peer support group

If you are alone on a placement make sure you have arranged a network of people you can contact if you need support. The peer group is seen by students as the second most important relationship after the supervisory relationship (Wallis and Hutchings, 1990) and can provide strong support for you when you are on fieldwork placement. Some of your colleagues might be working on placement in the same, or in a nearby service. A meeting with them once a week would enable you to share your experiences. You might even identify a topic or a theme to help focus your discussions. If there are several of you, you might ask someone to facilitate the group discussion. Some peer groups become **closed groups** where the membership is restricted. A closed group can provide a safe atmosphere for sharing issues of concern. In these groups you need to guard against supporting each other's weaknesses and focus instead on strengths. You also need to be positive and facilitate the development of new ideas and different ways of working.

4. YOUR PSYCHOLOGICAL NEEDS

There are many sorts of needs which you must consider when you are preparing yourself for fieldwork education, including psychological needs. Professional literature refers to states of anxiety, stress and burnout so we are going to examine these factors here and provide suggestions for recognizing and dealing with them.

Becoming anxious

Anxiety is very common and most students experience it at some time or another, and particularly before going on placement (Greenstein, 1983). Of course you may not experience anxiety at all, but if you do it is likely to relate to concerns about how you think you will function on placement, or how you think you are actually functioning once you are there. You might have perceptions about how the placement will affect personal relationships, how much support you will have or how well you feel accepted and included in the placement. Each factor can alter the state of your feelings. In this book we suggest various ways in which you can take control and actively prepare yourself for your fieldwork experience. Putting effort into thorough preparation should help allay any anxiety you feel. In order that you can recognize anxiety, we are going to explain it in a little more detail.

Anxiety is a state that is difficult to define. Anxiety might be described as a range of reactions from mere feelings of apprehension to feelings of complete panic. At the panic level, anxiety can be very debilitating, but if it is kept within normal limits it can become a motivating force which will provide you with the necessary impetus for learning and for adjusting to new situations. An old dictionary definition (Funk and Wagnalls, 1929) suggests that anxiety is a disturbance of mind regarding some uncertain event, indicating that it can be provoked by external factors. More recent definitions such as that in Roper (1987) describe anxiety as feelings of fear, apprehension or dread, thus explaining how it is experienced. Although it is an emotional response, anxiety is characterized by physiological symptoms which are outlined in Table 8.2.

Table 8.2 Signs and symptoms of anxiety

- increase in heart rate and cardiac output
- contraction of the blood vessels of the skin and intestines so that blood is diverted to the heart and lungs (pallor and loss of appetite)
- increase in muscle tone which is experienced as tension
- mobilization of blood sugar or glucose from the liver to provide energy
- dilation of the pupils
- goose flesh
- sweating, particularly on the palms, soles and axillae
- contraction of bladder and bowels with relaxation of their sphincter muscles

Source: Sainsbury, M. (1980) *Key to Psychiatry*, 3rd edn, Australia and New Zealand Book Company, Sydney.

Tiredness

There are several obvious reasons why you might become tired during your fieldwork placement. The demands of a different environment, travel and living conditions, meeting strangers and working in a place where you will also be assessed, all put pressure on you. Working with clients when you are not quite sure what you are doing but wanting to give your best professionally can also be wearing. You will find that your emotional responses to these situations burn up your energy. Many of these factors taken singly seem insignificant, but when they occur together they can raise your level of anxiety.

When you are in a strange environment you are not always able to manage your time efficiently. It may take you a long time to do things that are new to you. You will have to balance the time needed for thorough preparation with that needed for actually getting things done. It is important to realize this limitation and to accept that you may not be able to work as efficiently at first as you believe you should.

Your need for a quiet time

What can you do if you find yourself getting anxious or feeling stressed? Even though you think you are coping well your senses are being assaulted with new experiences, both physical and mental. You need time to absorb these experiences, to reflect on your ideas and your feelings. We suggest you set some time aside each day for a quiet time. It may occur at any time in the day, but try to schedule it when you will not be interrupted. Spending time in this way is quite acceptable and can be beneficial as a way of both relaxing and of consolidating learning.

Tips for dealing with high anxiety levels.

These are some of the things that you can do to help yourself manage your anxiety.

- Try to pinpoint the cause of your problem and plan a strategy for dealing with it.
- Accept personal responsibility for seeking the solution.
- Realize your problems are not unique.
- Sit or lie down, close your eyes and try to eliminate outside noise.
- Try to breathe slowly and to say to yourself 'I can handle this.'
- Massage your temples or the back of your neck or ask someone else to do it for you.

Your need to be in touch with your family

For some placements you might be away from home and at a distance from your family. Your ability to cope will depend on your personality and your life experience. You might be quite self-sufficient and enjoy the freedom of being independent but you might also find being away from home quite difficult. If you think you will miss those you are close to, try to think of ways in which you can keep in touch. Even taking photographs with you can help.

Your need to manage your personal problems

Trying to manage personal problems and placement problems at the same time can cause worry and anxiety. Remember that you will be working with clients who often have quite major problems. You may find that a client's problems mirror your own and this may make your reactions more severe. Sometimes events happen on placement which resurrect memories from the past. For example, you might find yourself dealing with the death of a client which brings back memories of the death of someone close to you. Alternatively you might find yourself working with a client with learning difficulties, or with someone who is having mental health problems similar to those experienced by a family member or a friend. If you know of anything in your life that could potentially be disturbing for you then share it with your educator. He or she may be more selective about the clients you work with or recommend strategies to help you come to terms with working with such clients. The decision to share this sort of information with your educator is quite personal, however, and one which you alone must make.

Changing anxiety into stress and burnout

You can see that there are circumstances which can potentially cause anxiety levels to rise. If you cannot control this anxiety you might find that it builds up too much and you enter a stage of stress. Your body responds by adapting to your chronically anxious state through your nervous or hormonal systems. Your heart rate alters, blood pressure rises and other changes occur in your bodily functions. The signs and symptoms of stress are outlined in Table 8.3.

If the signs and symptoms of stress are ignored or left unattended they will lead to the phenomenon known as **burnout**

Burnout

It is very unlikely that you will experience burnout as a student. Awareness of work-related stress helps you to avoid it or to deal with it quickly if you find it happening to you. We do think that it is important to describe burnout though as it is a serious condition. You might encounter it at some time in your professional life either in people you work with on placement or later when qualified. If anyone is suffering from burnout their remarks and reactions could have an effect on you. You might not understand the reasons behind the things they say or the things they do, particularly in relation to professional matters. The implications can be serious.

Burnout is an unpleasant phenomenon which is characterized by different stages which are even more distressing than anxiety and stress. Often burnout is characterized by negative views about the profession or the place of work. People suffering from burnout often start coming in late to work. They work ineffectively or even unsafely. They may be actively resistant to any forms of change and even may appear to dislike the clients and may make derogatory remarks about them. Some people feel trapped in their duties. They may feel that their job is boring and that they have little support and no understanding from others. They may also feel that they are not making any meaningful contribution to the job. Conversely, they may try too hard and have totally unrealistic expectations of themselves.

Recognizing phases of burnout

There are three phases of burnout that a person may experience. The first is characterized by physical and emotional exhaustion which can manifest itself in any of the following ways: tiredness in the morning, memory blocks, feelings of frustration or self-righteousness, finding fault with, or constantly blaming others, and loss of a sense of humour.

Table 8.3 Signs and symptoms of stress

Body signals	*Behavioural signals*	*Mental and emotional signals*
(How your body responds to stressors)	(How you act in response to stressors)	(How you think or feel in response to stressors)
Increase in, or loss of, appetite	Nervous tic or nervous habit, such as nail biting or tapping one's fingers or feet	Sense of loss of control
Nausea, indigestion or upset stomach		Loss of motivation (you feel like giving up)
Dry mouth	Restlessness or pacing	Worry, feeling of dread
Muscle tension		
Increased perspiration	Increased smoking, eating or drinking	Anxiety, nervousness
Headache from tension	Irritability or short temper	Change in mood
Constipation or diarrhoea	Too much sleep or loss of sleep	Loss of sex drive
Fatigue	Jaw clenching	Increased desire to smoke, eat or drink
Rash or skin irritation	Crying	Despair, sadness or hopelessness
Facial blushing or paling	Withdrawing from social contacts	Inability to enjoy life
Cold hands and/or feet	Depending on such medications as tranquillizers and pain pills	Difficulty in concentrating
Shortness of breath or rapid breathing		Feeling defensive

Therapy
Source: The American Occupational Therapy Association (1989).

	Points (circle if applicable)	How long? Weeks 1	Months 2	Over a year 3	How often? Sometimes 1	Frequently 2	Constantly 3	How intense? Mild 1	Moderate 2	Severe 3
Physical symptoms										
Fatigue	2									
Insomnia	3									
Headache	2									
Backache	1									
GI problems	2									
Weight loss/gain	1									
Shortness of breath	1									
Lingering cold	2									
Personal										
Bored	3									
Restless	2									
Stagnating	3									
Rationalizing	4									
Feeling indispensible	5									
Obsessed	5									
Depressed	3									
Behavioural										
Irritable	4									
Unable to enjoy or compliment colleagues success	4									
Cynical	5									
Defensive	4									
Faultfinding	4									
Dependence on alcohol	5									
Dependence on drugs	5									
Score	____									
					Grand total ____					

Directions

1. Add up the points for each symptom you circle

2. In the section that asks 'How long' add one point if you've had the symptom for weeks or two for months and three if over a year

3. In the second column, add one point if you experience symptoms sometimes, two if frequently, and three if you've had symptoms for more than one year

Rate the intensity of your symptoms with one point for mild, two for moderate and three for severe

Totals

20 – 25 : Possible problem, if marks are primarily in the physical category, could be a health problem

57 – 103 : Definite problem with work and attitude, especially if marks are fairly equally distributed among all categories

About to enter danger zone, professional treatment recommended

Figure 8.3 Check your own burnout potential. Reprinted with permission from *Medical Economics Magazine,* copyright © 1981

Source: from Halenar, J. (Senior Associate Editor) (1981) Doctors don't have to burn out. *Medical Economics Magazine,* Medical Economics Company.

The second phase is more serious. A person in this stage develops negative, cynical and often dehumanized attitudes about clients and other staff members. Clients are often referred to as if they were objects, they might not be referred to by name or even be introduced to you. Those who suffer from burnout often display anger and irritation, become rigid and inflexible or stubborn and they may become impotent. They display a sense of powerlessness, hopelessness and weariness, and they just want to be left alone.

The third phase is referred to as **terminal burnout** which is marked by complete and utter boredom on the job, cynicism about everything including work, home, others and self. At this stage those suffering from burnout might even become psychotic.

Because of the seriousness of the consequences of burnout, if you suspect that someone might be suffering from burnout and it is affecting your work then it would be advisable to speak to your fieldwork educator about it. If this course of action is not appropriate then we think it is better to contact someone at university and ask their advice. In case you need to check your potential for symptoms of burnout we have included a list for reference.

Finally, before we consider your physical needs on placement we would like you to think about 'letting go' both at the end of the day and also at the end of the placement.

Letting go

If you continue to live at home while on fieldwork placement then the problem of loneliness is less likely to arise. However, many students on placement find themselves in strange rooms, in a strange environment, and with people they do not know. From the discussions about stress and burnout it is easy to see how you might fall into the trap of studying in the evenings and shutting yourself away from people. This is not good for you. You need to get the balance of your work and social life into perspective. It is important to share some of your free time with others, to go out and enjoy yourself, and to do things that are not connected with your work. Be warned, however, when you are out with friends take care not to talk about your clients in public places. Your conversations can be overheard and clients can be identified by even simple descriptions. This breaks all the rules of confidentiality. On social occasions, leave work behind and just aim to have a good time. Celebrate the end of your placement and be sure not to take any problems away with you when you leave.

5. YOUR PHYSICAL HEALTH NEEDS

The state of your physical health contributes directly to the success of your placement and you should not take this for granted. Maintaining good health through a good diet and regular exercise will help you to cope with the normal stresses of the fieldwork experience and other things such as infections, that you might be exposed to. Taking responsibility for your own health and wellÔbeing is both a personal and professional matter. It is your responsibility to inform your fieldwork educator if you have health related problems which might affect your performance, such as back problems, fits, diabetes, or any kind of sensory problem. Being open about the problems will help the fieldwork educator manage both your needs and client needs safely.

Being vaccinated

In some placements, and particularly placements abroad, you may find yourself at risk of being exposed to certain communicable diseases. You must find out if it is necessary to have any particular vaccination. Usually your university will let you know what the requirements are but do not take this for granted. The diseases which you must be protected against before going on any fieldwork placement in the UK minimally are TB, hepatitis B, poliomyelitis and tetanus. Consult your family doctor if you cannot remember when you had the last dose of a particular vaccine. You may need a booster. Always ask if there are side effects and how long the immunity will last.

If you should go abroad, certain countries require evidence of vaccinations or other prophylactic measures taken before you arrive, such as tablets for malaria. Your general practitioner, a travel clinic or the relevant embassy of the country you are visiting should have all this information. Obtaining some of these vaccinations can take time so it is advisable to make arrangements well in advance.

Exceptions

If you belong to a religious order or follow a particular alternative health orientation which does not believe in having vaccinations then you may find yourself in a vulnerable and difficult position. Not only must you communicate this fact to the fieldwork coordinator at your university but you might need to take legal advice about this before you go on placement. We do not address these needs in the book as they are specific to each individual.

HIV/AIDS and other infectious diseases

On certain placements you might be exposed to clients who are HIV positive, who carry the AIDS virus or who have other infectious diseases. In the UK, guidelines are issued by a Advisory Committee on Dangerous Pathogens (ACDP). These are compiled for the Health and Safety Commission and the Health Departments and they are revised regularly. The counter infection measures that are presently accepted for those exposed to HIV and also to the virus of Hepatitis B are listed in Table 8.4 below.

Illness on placement

If you become ill while you are on your placement you should take remedial steps as ill health can affect you both personally and academically. This means taking

Table 8.4 Counterinfection measures against HIV exposure

- Preventing puncture wounds, cuts and abrasions in the presence of blood and body fluids and protecting against wounds, skin lesions, conjunctivae and mucosal surfaces.
- Applying simple protective measure designed to avoid contamination of the person or clothing and using good basic hygiene practices including regular handwashing.
- Controlling surface contamination by blood and body fluids by contaminent and disinfection.
- Avoiding the use of sharps (needles, pointed instruments, glassware etc.) whenever possible but when their use is essential, exercising particular care in handling and disposal.
- Disposing of clinical and other contaminated waste safely

responsibility for your own health (and possibly the health of others) by taking time out to recuperate and seeking medical advice as necessary. Nobody benefits from you persevering with fieldwork when you are unwell.

If you do become ill and miss several days, then you will find that your university has rules about the production of certificates and about making up lost time. If you are following a part-time programme and are an employee, you must fulfil the requirements of your workplace regarding the production of sickness certificates. No student should be disadvantaged in their academic programme by a temporary period of sickness. Although placement requirements still have to be fulfilled before you qualify, arrangements can normally be made to reschedule fieldwork later in the academic programme or to extend a period of fieldwork to enable you to make up lost hours. You will need to negotiate this with your tutors at university.

Back care

Back problems account for a large proportion of employee sickness in health services each year. As health professionals involved in the manual lifting and handling of clients it is essential that you understand the principles of back care and learn how to protect your back from injury. It is important to know, for instance, when it is safe to move a client single-handed, when the help of another person should be sought and when you must use a lifter (hoist) to transfer a client from one place to another.

Most universities will ensure that you have had some instruction in lifting and handling techniques before you go to your fieldwork placement. Some placements, however, take place very early in the academic programme and training may not be provided before the fieldwork experience. You must speak to your educator about any limitations in your knowledge.

The regulations which currently apply in the workplace are the Manual Handling Operations Regulation 1992 which place a statutory duty on employers to avoid unnecessary risk of harm to employees from any manual handling operations and to provide training for employees on how to handle loads correctly. As a student on placement you would be in the same position as an employee. Both you and your fieldwork educator have a responsibility to ensure that you know how to lift clients safely, using lifting devices where necessary. If you are unsure about lifting clients you must speak to your educator before participating in any manual lifting procedure. You have a duty of care to the client and your colleagues not to put them at risk, and you have a duty to yourself to look after your back and learn to lift correctly.

SUMMARY

In this chapter we have stressed the importance of understanding yourself and recognizing your personal needs before and during the fieldwork experience. This knowledge and awareness, particularly in relation to attitudes, values and beliefs will help you in your preparations for fieldwork and enable you to deal effectively with issues as they arise. Ways of avoiding anxiety and stress, and of recognizing burnout, have been presented. Emphasis has been placed on thorough preparation for fieldwork, including identifying support mechanisms on which to draw during the experience.

Many students take short cuts in preparing for their placement and fail to think about themselves and their needs, particularly their intra-personal or psychological needs. This chapter has highlighted those areas which require special attention to help you cope with the demands of the fieldwork experience.

REFERENCES

AOTA (1987) *Fieldwork evaluation for the occupational therapist*. The American Occupational Therapy Association Inc., MD.

AOTA (1989) *Understanding stress: strategies for a healthier mind and body*. The American Occupational Therapy Association, Inc., MD.

Barker, L. L. (1987) *Communication*, 4th edn. Prentice Hall Inc., New Jersey.

Boud, D., Cohen, R. and Walker, D. (eds) (1985) *Reflection: Turning Experience Into Learning*. Kogan Page, New York.

Brust, P. L. (1986) Student burnout: the clinical instructor can spot it and manage it. *Clinical Management in Physiotherapy*, **6**(3), 18–21.

Cohn, E. (1993) Fieldwork education: applying theory to practice. In H. Hopkins and H. Smith (eds), *Willard and Spackman's Occupational Therapy*, 8th edn. J.B. Lippincott, Philadelphia.

Fleming, M. H. (1994) in Mattingly, C. and Fleming, M. H., *Clinical Reasoning: Forms of Inquiry in a Therapeutic Practice*. F.A. Davis Company, Philadelphia.

Frum, D. C. and Opacich, K. J. (1987) *Supervision: Development of Therapeutic Competence*. American Occupational Therapy Association Inc. and Rush University, MD.

Funk and Wagnalls Dictionary (1929) *Desk Standard Dictionary of the English Language*. Funk & Wagnalls Co., New York.

Greenstein, L. R. (1983) Student anxiety toward Level 11 Fieldwork. *American Journal of Occupational Therapy*, **37**(2), 89–95.

Henry, J. N. (1985) Using feedback and evaluation effectively in clinical supervision. *Physical Therapy*, **65**(3), 354–7.

Ilott, I. (1988) *Failure: The Clinical Supervisor's Perspective*. Unpublished M.Ed dissertation, University of Nottingham, England.

Javernick, J. A. (1994) Professional growth through mentoring. *OT Week*, **8** (24), 16 June 1994.

Loganbill, C., Hardy, E. and Delworth, U. (1982) Supervision: a conceptual model. *Counseling Psychologist*, **10**(1), 3–42.

Luft, J. (1969) *Of Human Interaction.* National Press Books. Palo Alto, California.

Mattingly, C. (1994) in Mattingly, C. and Fleming, M. *Clinical Reasoning: Forms of Inquiry in a Therapeutic Practice.* F.A. Davis Company, Philadelphia.

Muldary, T. (1983) *Burnout and Health Professionals: Manifestations and Management.* Appleton-Century-Crofts. Norwalk, CN.

Robertson, S. C. (1994) Mentorship: it's not just a job, it's a guiding light. *CAN-AM Courier*, Boston.

Roper, N. (ed.)(1987) *Pocket Medical Dictionary*, 14th edn. Churchill Livingstone, Edinburgh.

Sainsbury, M. J. (1980) *Key to Psychiatry*, 3rd edn. Australian and New Zealand Book Company, Sydney.

Schon, D. (1987) *Educating the Reflective Practitioner.* Jossey Bass, San Francisco.

Schwartz, K (1984) An approach to supervision of students on fieldwork. *American Journal of Occupational Therapy*, **38**(6), 393–7.

Schwartzberg S. (1992) *Self-disclosure and empathy in occupational therapy.* Paper presented at the Occupational Therapy Conference, Trinity College, Dublin, Ireland; July 1992.

Wallis, D. and Hutchings, S. (1990) The attainment of professional attitudes: the use of group based work in a clinical and school based setting. *British Journal of Occupational Therapy*, **53**(2), 48–52.

Weimer, R. (1994) *Student transition from academic to fieldwork settings.* In *Guide to Fieldwork Education.* American Occupational Therapy Association, pp. 171–7.

Young, M. and Quinn, E. (1992) *Theories and Principles of Occupational Therapy.* Churchill Livingstone, Edinburgh.

Yuen, H. K (1990) Fieldwork students under stress. American Journal of Occupational Therapy, **44**(1), 80–1.

9 Taking responsibility

This chapter covers:

- students' responsibilities before, during and at the end of the placement;
- procedural, practical and educational activities which should be undertaken for effective participation in fieldwork education.

In this chapter we encourage you to take responsibility for preparing yourself for the fieldwork experience. Often an active approach can help you to feel more in control and, as we pointed out in the last chapter, being proactive can lessen your anxiety and help you to feel more prepared for the fieldwork situation. You will often see words like **autonomous** and **proactive** in the professional literature. These words suggest taking individual responsibility and being forward thinking. This chapter will encourage you to take initiative and to plan ahead. It will focus on the things that you can do before, during and after your placement. The chapter is in three sections.

Section 1 examines responsibilities before your placement.

Section 2 examines responsibilities during your placement.

Section 3 examines responsibilities at the end of your placement.

Each part is subdivided into three subsections: procedural activities, practical activities and educational activities which should guide you as you prepare for, participate in, and evaluate fieldwork.

1. RESPONSIBILITIES BEFORE YOUR PLACEMENT

Procedural activities

One of the things that you must do before going on placement is to communicate with your fieldwork educator. Your fieldwork coordinator at university will inform you about the procedure to follow. You may be expected to write a letter or complete a specific form and send it to your fieldwork educator. Once you have made contact with the placement you might receive another form to complete and return which asks for further personal information and details of your previous experience. When filling it in you should include any relevant experience you have had either before you started your Occupational Therapy course or during it. Give information about any voluntary work or professional work you have done, and provide details of placements you have completed. The fieldwork educator needs to have sufficient information to form an image of you and to facilitate the planning of the placement.

If there is no form then take responsibility and write to your fieldwork educator. Writing is better than telephoning. It allows you time to think about what you want to say and allows your educator to deal with it when convenient. When you write, ask your fieldwork educator to send you information about the placement including accommodation, parking facilities, catering and other environmental factors that are of specific relevance to you.

Practical activities

Much of what you need to do depends on where you are going for your placement, whether it is near your home (or where you normally stay) or away from home or in another country. Find out how to travel to the placement, and identify the exact building in which the service is based. Hospitals often comprise many buildings and it can take time to move from one part of the site to another. Ask what the normal working hours are as these vary. You can plan your journey and adjust the travelling time accordingly. This may sound rather basic but it is worth finding out well in advance. Factors such as rush hour traffic, trouble spots on certain routes, connections between trains and/or buses need to be identified. A good map of the area (also useful for home visits), details of travel routes and knowledge of parking sites are all things that you can obtain beforehand. A trial run before your first day will give you confidence about finding the place in good time.

Placements away

If you will be living away from your normal accommodation then you will need to find a place to stay. The placement may have a hostel, if not, then ask if there is a list of recommended lodging places. You need to be comfortable while working at the placement so you need to know what is available and what you need to take with you. Be prepared to take cutlery, crockery and essential cooking pans if you intend to cater for yourself.

Code of dress

One of the responsibilities that you have during your placement is to observe correctly the code of dress adopted for the service. Presentation is an important aspect of professional life and professional demeanour. This is referenced in the College of Occupational Therapists' Code of Ethics and Professional Conduct for Occupational Therapists (1995). Be sure that you find out about uniform requirements before you start the placement. Some hospitals require uniform to be worn, other placements permit casual dress. Take particular care with your footwear. Shoes need to support you well as you work on your feet all day. Open-toed sandals will not be allowed in any workshop. Flat shoes with non-slip soles will be required in most environments and will be essential in any setting where you will be lifting and moving clients.

The way you dress and present yourself makes a statement about you and about your profession. It is one of the most immediate things to be noticed by staff from all departments and by clients with whom you will work. It is important for you to be dressed in such a way that you fit in with staff and clients and that is practical for the work you will be doing. If there are discrepancies in the dress code of team members, take the lead from the occupational therapists and if you are still unsure, discuss the subject with your fieldwork educator. It is far better to have open discussion and clarify the situation than to be told that your mode of dress is unacceptable. Remember, it is not for you as a student to make decisions on the mode of dress, you must conform to the situation you are in.

It is also important to be sensitive about wearing jewellery and perfume. Both should be discreet. Necklaces, bracelets, earrings and some rings are not only inappropriate they can also present a safety risk to you, your colleagues and/or the clients.

Personal hygiene

One thing not often mentioned when discussing dress and presentation is personal hygiene. Remember that you will be working very close to clients so use deodorants and ensure that your dental care is thorough. It is embarrassing for both the student and the fieldwork educator if this issue has to be addressed during the placement.

Using your car

You should clarify whether a car is needed when placements are allocated. If you do not have access to a car then it may affect the experience you get. Even though you have a car you may choose not to use it for business purposes. You may not wish to take patients or clients in your vehicle, or your car might not be reliable enough for you to use for work purposes. Your expectations need to be clearly stated so that your fieldwork coordinator knows which placements to allocate to you, and so that the fieldwork educator knows how to plan for your fieldwork experience.

You will find that some placements, mostly those in the community, require you to have use of a car. Using your car for work undertaken for the fieldwork setting, for instance for home visits or travel between sites, is usually classed as 'business use' by insurance companies. If you elect to use your car for the official business of the placement you must be insured for this purpose. Your insurance company may be prepared to add this class of use to your policy for little or no extra cost. The fieldwork educator may wish to see written evidence of insurance cover before you undertake any journeys.

If you do use your car for business purposes you must clarify **in advance** who will pay for your petrol. Rarely does a service reimburse students for costs associated with journeys on duty, and neither does the university. This means that you may need to finance it yourself. You need to be very clear about whether you are willing to accept these costs.

Professional indemnity

Being insured at work is essential. If you are a student on a course in the UK you will be a student registrant with the British Association of Occupational Therapists which provides insurance cover while you are on placement provided that you are working under the supervision of an occupational therapist. If you are going abroad you may need separate insurance cover. The rules about professional indemnity vary from country to country. In some countries you will have to insure yourself privately in order to be protected. It is worth finding out if the insurance which you automatically have in your home country would cover you in the country in which you are planning to work. Other countries, such as Canada and the United States of America have strict rules about the work a student may, or may not, do with a client. You should take responsibility for asking about the conditions.

Consulting past students and information files

Sometimes the university fieldwork coordinator maintains files, possibly computerized, which give details of placements used. Some placements have a prospectus with information for students which is kept at the university for reference. Often students who have been to a particular service will update the material in the file and add their own comments about their experience of that placement. Files at the university are a good source of information but a word of advice – check the date of the latest information because not all files are as up to date as they might be. You could always contact a student who has been to that placement previously. Even if that student did not have a positive experience, you can still learn from his or her story. If this is the case, adopt a positive attitude and realize that good learning can occur in all situations (Weimer, 1994).

Placements abroad

If your fieldwork experience is to be in another country the person designated to supervise you while on placement should be able to provide you with details of the placement setting. It is obviously essential to plan well in advance. Correspondence by letter can take several days or even weeks. Use fax facilities if they are available, but seek guidance from your fieldwork educator about the best way to communicate. You will need to ask all the same questions about board and lodging, and you will need to state if you have any dietary or mobility requirements. Find out about the climate, the clothing and as much as possible about the local customs. An embassy can supply you with up to date details about the country in which you will be doing your placement.

You may need to ask about visas and about vaccinations, injections or other prophylactic measures, such as anti-malarial tablets, that might either be desirable or required for entry to the country. Ask if there will be access to medical facilities should you need them, and always give the placement full details of a contact person at home, even if you are not asked for this information.

Educational activities

Once you know where you are going on placement you can do a great deal to prepare yourself educationally for the experience and this will assist you to function in the placement and ultimately to learn from the experience. Sadly many students fail to see how these preparations may help. The fieldwork coordinator at the university will probably hold briefing sessions prior to the placement but these are often limited by time because of commitments to other aspects of the educational programme. You will get basic information and advice, but if you rely purely on this time for preparation you may be disadvantaged. The proposals in this section are intended to help you further.

Identifying your intent

According to Boud and Walker (1991) a truthful self-examination of your **intent** for the placement is important. What these authors mean by intent is asking yourself the question 'what do I hope to get out of this placement?' Your intent helps you to shape your experience. As we have said before, each situation is different and each placement offers different experiences. There may be other events in your life at the time of the placement which can affect the way you feel and perform, and which may influence your intent. There can therefore be different forms of intent at different times. Be honest with yourself as you approach the placement and examine all aspects which might have a bearing on how it will go.

The following are some examples of questions you might ask yourself or statements you might make in relation to your intent.

Questions:

- 'Why did I choose this placement?'
- 'Will I gain knowledge on this placement which will add to my existing knowledge?'

Statements:

- 'I thought it would be easy and wouldn't require much work.'
- 'I really enjoy working with ...'
- 'It's near my home so it won't be a problem to get there.'
- 'I want to find out more about ...'
- 'I've heard a lot about ... and thought I would get a great deal out of working with him/her.'

- 'I want to get away from home and this is a good excuse.'
- 'I've heard this is a good placement so I thought I'd like to try it.'

These are just a few examples of students' intent for choosing a placement. You can see that there could be many more. They divide roughly into those which relate directly to professional development and those that have nothing to do with it. You can also see how your intent can shape the whole of your experience so we suggest that you are clear and honest with yourself when you state your intent. In this way you will know how the outcome of the placement might be affected.

Examining your past experiences

Once you know the age group and the clients with whom you will be working it can be a good idea to list your past experiences of such clients or even those related to one individual. You might know someone in your family or a neighbour or a friend with a similar condition. Write down what you remember about how the condition has affected their life. This exercise broadens your thinking and enriches the experience (McKay and Ryan, 1995). You might also have seen patients portrayed in films, or have heard disabled people talk about their experiences on the radio or television. See what you can recall because this will give you a basis on which to build.

Examining your values

A value is often defined as a belief or an ideal to which an individual is committed. Values are central to shaping professional directions and behaviours (Engelhardt, 1986, cited in Fondiller *et al*., 1990). Values can be looked at from a personal perspective and from a professional perspective. As we pointed out in Chapter 8, an examination of your values can improve your awareness of the fieldwork experience.

Examining your formal knowledge base

As soon as you know the condition(s) of the clients that you are likely to be working with, you can look back at your lecture notes to see what relevant theoretical work you have covered. The World Health Organization (WHO) (1980) definitions of **impairment, disability** and **handicap** might help you to structure your thoughts. The WHO definitions are as follows:

Impairment	Any loss or abnormality of psychological, physiological or anatomical structure or function
Disability	Any restriction or lack of ability (resulting from impairment) to perform an activity in the manner or within the range considered normal for a human being
Handicap	A disadvantage for a given individual, resulting from an impairment or disability, that limits or prevents the fulfilment of a 'survival' role that is normal (depending on age, sex, social and cultural factors) for that individual.

As Turner *et al*. (1992) note, impairment is the loss or limitation of ability, disability is the effect such loss or limitation has on functional performance, and handicap is the restriction these limitations place on the person's lifestyle. Using this framework you might think about any case stories or studies you have done or any people you have known. You might additionally think whether you have any information about theoretical approaches or the types of assessments or interventions that might be used with such clients. Think about what work you have covered in the different study blocks, units or modules you have completed. Relevant information may come from many sources.

Do not attempt to memorize your notes, but try to visualize an integration of all the different components of your studies so that you begin to have a more comprehensive picture. In your mind's eye try to piece together any client experiences which you can recall, including any information on pathology. Put these together with relevant notes from anatomy and with anything you remember about medications used for such conditions, including side effects. Students tend to understand things better when they look at the person's problem first and then fit in the relevant bioscience afterwards. Integrating aspects of knowledge, 'putting it all together' (Slater, 1989) is something that students tend to find hard to do, especially during the placement when there are so many other distractions. You can take responsibility for doing these educational activities yourself. You should not need anyone else to help you unless you need anything clarifying.

Identifying practical skills

While you are sorting through your lecture notes it is a good idea to identify any practical skills which you think may be of use in the placement, and which you need to revise or learn. You may realize that you have acquired skills previously during fieldwork education which might be useful, although you may find that skills are applied differently in different placements. Remember that all work in therapy is bound by context. Certain ways of doing things go with certain placements, so be prepared to be flexible and to learn from the new context. You can always ask your fieldwork educator to explain any differences you perceive between one therapeutic environment and another.

Another useful activity before you start your placement is to practise skills on, or with, a friend. This should give you added confidence because you can gain immediate feedback from an informed source and perfect your technique at the same time (Ryan, 1995).

Searching the literature

Now is the best time to find out about the latest thinking and action in the field in which you will be practising. If you know how to do a library search for new books or recent articles, then do one and read the abstracts to select the ones likely to inform you best. If you cannot do an on-line search ask your librarian to show you how! Depending on your stage of development, you might wish to search wider than in the Occupational Therapy literature. You might like to explore literature in allied fields of study such as physiology, psychology or medicine, and to find out about current practice with such clients in other professions. There are many other sources of information which might be useful to tap into if you have time before your placement starts.

Reading

There is plenty of scope for reading around topics relevant to your placement. You may well be sent a recommended reading list by your fieldwork educator and clearly this is where you should start. The literature searches mentioned above could also produce relevant material. Unless prompted to do otherwise, give priority to the more up-to-date texts and articles. Time will always be a limiting factor but there are clear advantages to be gained from immersing yourself in literature to inform your fieldwork studies in the same way as you would for any academic studies. In fact it will help you to look at other perspectives on disability or on working with disabled or dysfunctional people. For example, you might look up the work of Sacks (1986; 1995) who offers valuable observational and reasoning insights from the perspective of a doctor. You might also read some personal accounts of responses to disability written by people who actually suffer from a condition. Keep texts to hand for your fieldwork so that you can use them as references during your placement.

Identifying your learning needs

You may well be sent a list of **Aims and Objectives** for the placement before you start. They sometimes appear as **Processes and Outcomes** or **Learning Opportunities**. Whatever the format, they will give you some idea of what the placement has to offer. If you have done some preparatory work you should be able to see where the gaps are in your knowledge and skills, and what your learning needs are likely to be. You may find it helpful to complete the cognitive knowledge check list (Higgs, 1990) in Table 9.1 to assess yourself in an informal way. The exercise could provide you with a starting point from which to negotiate your learning contract when you arrive at the placement. It will also indicate the amount of work which might be ahead of you and allow you to adjust to the demands of the placement.

We conclude this section with an overall checklist of things you can do before the placement starts (Table 9.2).

2. RESPONSIBILITIES DURING YOUR PLACEMENT

As in the previous section, the things that you should take responsibility for during your placement are listed under the same headings: procedural activities, practical activities and educational activities.

Table 9.1 Self-rating checklist for clinical reasoning

KEY
0 = Needs considerable improvement
1 = Needs some improvement
2 = Is adequate
3 = Is good
4 = Is very good

SKILL AREA	SELF-RATING
Collection of clinical data (perceptual and psychomotor skills)	
Interpersonal skills in data collection	
Interpersonal skills in decision-making	
Knowledge base (scope, content, relevance)	
Knowledge base (organization)	
Knowledge base (accessibility)	
Cognitive skills (reasoning, logic)	
Cognitive skills (intuition, lateral thinking, creative thinking)	
Cognitive skills (hypothesis generation and testing)	
Skills in critical evaluation and review	
Skills in metacognition	
Skills in critical self-evaluation	

Reprinted with permission.
Source: Higgs, J. (1990) Fostering the acquisition of clinical reasoning skills. *New Zealand Journal of Physiotherapy,* **12**, 13–17.

Procedural activities

Induction

An induction programme should be prepared for you by your fieldwork educator. This is discussed more thoroughly in Chapter 10. However, there are some activities for which you can take responsibility at the start of your placement. It is important to familiarize yourself with the actual procedures of the service and routines which will help you to feel part of the team. Find out about the procedures for entering the building, security and for signing in and out. Locate the notice boards and/or message books that staff use. Find out where the fire alarms, appliances and exits are located. Last but not least, find out what arrangements are made, and what facilities are available, for taking coffee and lunch breaks!

Professional responsibilities

Working to a Code of Ethics and Professional Conduct
Each national professional association has a Code of Ethics and Professional

Table 9.2 Checklist for activities before a placement

Before the placement communicate with your fieldwork educator:
- provide a full profile about yourself
- provide details of special requirements
- ask about accommodation
- find out exact locations and travel arrangements
- ask about the local environment
- ask about working hours
- find out about uniform requirements

For placements abroad:
- ask about best ways to communicate
- ask about board and lodging
- find out about visas
- ask about injections, vaccinations, tablets
- enquire about medical facilities/insurance
- give details of contact persons
- ask about insurance coverage
- find out about dress requirements

Transport enquiries:
- ask about the need for a car
- enquire about insurance for business use of the car
- clarify reimbursement for petrol usage

Placement experience:
- look at files kept in the university
- contact past students who have attended the placement

Educational preparation:
- ask how many hours are timetabled for briefing sessions at your university
- do a self-examination or 'intent' exercise
- examine your past experiences from all sources
- examine your values
- examine your formal knowledge base and try to make connections
- brush up on your practical skills
- tap into other professional sources of information
- make sure that your reading is up to date

Conduct which expresses the principles of practice in that country. You should take responsibility for finding out which Code is followed where you are working. Acceptance of those principles is a professional expectation. Professional behaviour is thus guided towards that which is commonly accepted as good practice.

The Code of Ethics and Professional Conduct for Occupational Therapists (1995) is in existence in the UK to provide

> a public statement of the values and principles used in promoting and maintaining high standards of professional behaviour in Occupational Therapy... The Code provides directions for occupational therapists and may be used by others to determine the standards of professional conduct which can be expected from occupational therapists and students (p. 3).

A breach of the Code in practice is treated very seriously, both for students and for qualified staff. Educational programmes leading to Occupational Therapy qualification normally require the Code to be respected. Explicit procedures for dealing with breaches of the Code may be part of the programme regulations.

As professional practice becomes more complex there is increasing concern about ethical issues such as cost containment (Neuhaus, 1988) and practice dilemmas (Hansen, Kamp and Reitz 1988). Barnitt (1993) argues that ethics teaching should be integrated into professional studies at university as part of the preparations for practice. Discussions on ethical dilemmas can increase awareness of ethical problems which might be encountered. It will obviously be helpful if you have participated in discussions about ethical dilemmas or have read up about ethical principles before you embark on fieldwork education. Any ethical issues which become apparent to you on placement can then be addressed in an informed way.

Relating to the team

When working with team members you must demonstrate respect for the role that each plays in client care. The role that members of different professions perform varies from team to team so do not assume that you know. Check who takes responsibility for what, especially where roles appear to be blurred. This will help you to clarify your role within the team.

A chart identifying team members, their responsibilities and the organizational or hierarchical relationship between key people will help you to become aware of relationships. If you are not given one, try to draw one for yourself. The dynamics of the team can affect behaviour, performance, and ultimately service delivery. You will need to become aware of team dynamics and work with them, or at least within the constraints of them. Note who talks a lot, who breaks the tension in awkward moments, who has a tendency to be aggressive, who facilitates team efforts and who compromises. This may help you to see the influence that different members have on the team.

Your presence can change team dynamics so you also need to be sensitive to the consequences of your behaviour. Noticing the behavioural responses of your colleagues can help you to become aware of your own behaviour and its effects on others. This can help as you adjust in the new situation.

Educational activities

Responsibility for learning

The learning contract is a more formal agreement which identifies your specific learning needs and how they will be met. The contract helps structure and guide your work. It should be referred to frequently and modified as necessary. You should take responsibility personally for following it through. We address this in detail in Chapter 10. Taking responsibility for learning means becoming actively engaged in your fieldwork experience. As Boud and Walker (1991) suggest, the more actively you are engaged the greater the likelihood that the event can be a significant learning experience. Be alert to learning opportunities and be proactive in taking advantage of them. Do not wait until you are directed; have ready a well-thought-out action plan for achieving your goals.

Responsibility with clients

We discussed earlier the ways in which you could take responsibility for planning and for finding out about the client group with which you expect to work during your placement. Even if you are unfamiliar with the therapeutic area remember that you are working with people and not conditions (Peloquin, 1993). Take responsibility for talking with clients and with their families and carers. Find out about their individual interests and what brings meaning to their lives. If you do this informally you will become much more adept in more formal interviews.

In the literature, making meaning out of a client's story is a major component of **narrative reasoning** (Mattingly, 1991) and was a focus of clinical reasoning studies with occupational therapists in the 1980s. The ability to **empathize** with people you work with is a highly developed skill (Schwartzberg, 1992) and one that needs constant attention and refinement. You will find that the more you relate to individuals as people, the more the therapeutic intervention will become clear. Too often students are concerned about the procedural aspects of the work – what assessments to do, what interventions to plan – that they forget about interactional aspects. Fleming and Mattingly (1994) called this 'the underground practice' because previously its importance was not openly and overtly acknowledged.

Dreyfus and Dreyfus (1986) identified that students, especially in the early stages of their education, fail to see the situation as a whole and just see different factors as separate entities. If you have an action plan that incorporates the more 'human' side of your work this will help you to develop your practice in a more holistic way. Your fieldwork educator should help you to develop these skills.

Confidentiality

One other responsibility that you must take for yourself is that of respecting the confidentiality of the people with whom you are working. This is addressed specifically in the Code of Ethics and Professional Conduct for Occupational Therapists (1995). You should avoid talking about clients in public places. Even if you do not identify someone by name, a description of their circumstances can identify the person. Written material with information about clients should be carefully stored, especially if the material is to be used for academic work beyond the fieldwork setting. Total anonymity is required, so all references which might identify a client or the service must be erased. Tippex or whitener is often inadequate for the job because details can often be seen if the paper is held up to light. A breach of confidentiality is a serious disciplinary offence for all employees, including students, and will be dealt with as such.

Ending a therapeutic relationship

When you leave your placement, you will need to end the therapeutic relationship with any client you have been working with. This is a very important process but there is little mention of this in research studies either from the therapist's or client's perspective. Nevertheless, it is a process requiring a responsible and sensitive approach.

Clients receiving health care must know that you are a student and they have a right to refuse to work with you (Patient's Charter, 1991). Normally people do not object but since they know that you are a student they should realize that you are not a permanent member of staff, and that your time with them will be limited. Do not take this for granted, however, make it clear in your initial discussions so that the person has a sense of the time involved. As you near the end of the placement, raise the issue with the client, say that you will be leaving at the end of the following week and give him or her an idea of what will happen once you are gone. Tell the client who is taking over his or her care, arrange for introductions if necessary, and for an overlap of work in the last week wherever possible. The client should then be prepared for the change of therapeutic arrangements.

Many aspects of therapy cause personal feelings to be expressed and if you have been empathetic with a client you will find that you have been drawn into that person's life. This obviously depends on the circumstances but it is an inevitability of practice. No longer is it considered professional to be absolutely objective and uninvolved, it is all a matter of degree. This is why, in some areas of practice, and particularly in mental health, supervision is provided on a regular basis. It helps to keep things in perspective. One of the main objectives in Occupational Therapy is that of independence, and you need to encourage this in your clients rather than allowing them to become dependent on you. This has particular relevance when you leave the placement. An advantage of working in a team is that intervention need not always take place with one person, there are others around to share the client's care.

Balancing your life and flowing with it

One of the major tenets of Occupational Therapy is that of **balance**. It is a factor that we search for in our clients, and we work with them towards achieving this goal. We look for a balance between the time they spend on personal care, work and leisure activities. The same applies in life for any of us. When you are on your placement you must consider balance in your life and take responsibility for it. Even though you might be fascinated with your work you must allow yourself time to relax and to meet friends socially. Another theory, that of flow theory (Csikszentmihalyi, 1993) conversely suggests that if you are working intently and deriving positive feelings of happiness and 'flow' from this activity then the amount of actual time spent doing it is irrelevant. If you are thoroughly and positively immersed in your learning experience then go along with it and it will not be harmful to your health. You must, however, achieve a healthy balance of work and social activity in your own way. To conclude this section, Table 9.3 provides a checklist for activities while you are on placement.

3. RESPONSIBILITIES AT THE END OF, AND AFTER, YOUR PLACEMENT

Procedural and practical activities

Feedback

Normally there is a feedback or evaluation form for the placement which you should fill out before you leave. The purpose of this form is to give information to the service

Table 9.3 Checklist for activities on a placement

During the placement:

- find out about the security procedures in existence
- locate notice boards and message books
- look for fire alarms and exits
- buy deodorants and appropriate dental cleansers
- be familiar with the appropriate code of professional conduct
- become familiar with expected roles
- find out about the organization
- be perceptive about team interactions
- be aware of your presence and your behaviour
- be alert to learning opportunities
- talk informally to the clients and **listen** to them
- think about confidentiality issues

about your total fieldwork experience; it is a quality assurance measure. Like any other type of feedback, it is a formal way of evaluating the fieldwork placement and the fieldwork educator. It may be the only formal opportunity you have for giving feedback. It is also the vehicle that enables change and growth to take place in the placement, but this will depend on how you write your feedback.

Feedback may be favourable or unfavourable, but it needs to be constructive. It never helps to be judgemental, it does help if you provide an example of how aspects of the placement may be improved. Below are two examples of feedback statements, one of which is unhelpful and the other which is constructive. You should always strive to provide feedback which is constructive so that the recipient becomes aware of both the problem and the suggestion for change.

A critical, unhelpful statement

'Inadequate and irregular supervision'.

A constructive, precise statement

'Although I appreciate that you were extremely busy, it would have been helpful to have supervision scheduled at a regular time each week instead of having to snatch it between meetings.'

Normally you should wait until **after** you have received your assessment, or formal evaluation, before you give this form to your educator. Sometimes students post the form back after they leave. This avoids confrontation but it does not allow the opportunity for discussion. You also need to gain practice in giving constructive criticism as part of your professional development, so we recommend that you hand the feedback form in personally at the end of your last day, and be prepared to discuss it if necessary. As with any professional report you should complete your feedback form with care. You should be aware that some academic settings ask for a copy of the feedback form for their files. Check who should have a copy, and be sure to keep one for yourself.

On a more informal note, many students write thank you letters or cards to their fieldwork educator after they leave, both as a courtesy and as an acknowledgement of the effort that has gone into planning and providing the placement. These letters are usually much appreciated.

Educational activities at the end of the placement

Reports

Some academic settings require students to present written reports, essays or some form of appraisal of the placement. The fieldwork educator may be asked to verify the accuracy of information in the report which is then marked by university staff. Students often give, or send a copy of the finished report to the placement to be kept as a reference.

Returning to the academic setting

In her article about the differences between the academic and the clinical setting Cohn (1993) writes about the transition from the classroom to the clinic. What is not mentioned in literature, however, is the return from the clinic to the classroom. Many students report a feeling of deflation; they often want to continue working in practice. Students also report a feeling of strangeness with their peers. They have often had profound experiences where a great deal of professional growth has taken place. This can be difficult to explain and share. Disorientation can take a few weeks to overcome and it is perfectly natural. One way of looking at this phenomenon is to consider it as part of the grieving process; it requires a 'letting go'. Being aware of this reaction can be very helpful and can enable you to cope with your feelings.

Debriefing and reflection

The fieldwork coordinator will normally allocate time for debriefing back at university, but as for briefing sessions prior to the placement, debriefing sessions are often very short. Nevertheless they are an extremely important conclusion to the fieldwork experience and one which allows for further learning. Kolb (1984) emphasizes the importance of reflecting on the experience you have just had. He believes that, unless you undertake this reflection, deep learning is less likely to occur. Personal reflection on fieldwork is a responsibility you should take very seriously so that you gain as much as you can from the learning opportunities you have.

Finally, Table 9.4 provides a checklist of those activities which are important as you complete the placement.

SUMMARY

This chapter has outlined various activities you can carry out to help you prepare for the placement and conduct yourself professionally while you are there. They include communicating with your fieldwork educator, finding out in advance about the placement setting, taking stock of and enhancing your skills and knowledge base

Table 9.4 Checklist for activities at completion of placement

At the end of your placement:

- let your clients know when you will be leaving
- let your clients know who will be taking over working with them and arrange for an overlap in work
- seek supervision if you have difficulties leaving a client
- make sure that all the paperwork is up to date
- fill in the feedback form in a constructive manner and give specific examples
- write a 'thank you' letter or card
- complete any written work for the university
- send a copy of the written work to the placement for reference
- reflect on and thoroughly prepare your verbal or written feedback to your peers at university
- listen carefully and question others' experience

as a preparation for practice. Particular features of the Code of Ethics and Professional Conduct are highlighted, such as maintaining professional demeanour and confidentiality while gaining fieldwork experience. Responsibilities at the end of the placement are also explained such as 'letting go' and providing feedback on the experience.

REFERENCES

Barnitt, R. (1993) Deeply troubling questions; the teaching of ethics in undergraduate courses. *British Journal of Occupational Therapy*, **56**(11), 401–6.

Boud, D. and Walker, D. (1991) *Experience and Learning; Reflection at Work.* Deakin University Press, Geelong, Victoria.

Cohn, E. (1993) *Fieldwork Education; Applying Theory to Practice.* In H. Hopkins and H. Smith (eds), *Willard and Spackman's Occupational Therapy*, 8th edn, J.B. Lippincott, Philadelphia.

College of Occupational Therapists (1995) *Code of Ethics and Professional Conduct for Occupational Therapists.* College of Occupational Therapists, London.

Csikszentmihalyi, M. (1993) Activity and happiness: towards a science of occupation. *Occupational Science: Australia*, 1(1), 38–42.

Dreyfus, H and Dreyfus, S. (1986) *Mind over Machine; the Power of Human Intuition and Expertise in the Era of the Computer.* The Free Press, New York.

Engelhardt, H. T. (1986) The importance of values in shaping professional direction and behaviour: occupational therapy education. In *Target 2000. Proceedings of a Conference on Promoting Excellence in Education*, 39–44, Rockville MD. The American Occupational Therapy Association. In E. Fondiller, L. Rosage, B. Neuhaus (1990) Values influencing clinical Reasoning in occupational therapy: an exploratory study. *Occupational Therapy Journal of Research*, **10**(1), 41–55.

Fleming, M. and Mattingly, C. (1994) Giving language to practice. In *Clinical Reasoning – Forms of Inquiry in a Therapeutic Practice*, F.A. Davis Company, Philadelphia.

Hansen R., Kamp, L. and Reitz, S. (1988) Two practitioners analyses of occupational therapy practice dilemmas. *American Journal of Occupational Therapy*, **42**(5), 312–19.

Higgs, J. (1990) Fostering the acquisition of clinical reasoning skills. *New Zealand Journal of Physiotherapy*, **18**, 13–17.

Kolb, D. A. (1984) *Experiential Learning*. Prentice Hall Inc., Englewood Cliffs, New Jersey.

Mattingly, C. (1991) The narrative nature of clinical reasoning. *American Journal of Occupational Therapy*, **45**(11), 998–1005.

McKay, E. and Ryan, S. (1995) Clinical reasoning through story telling: examining a student's case story on a fieldwork placement. *British Journal of Occupational Therapy*, **58**(6), 234–8.

Neuhaus, B. (1988) Ethical considerations in clinical reasoning: the impact of technology on cost containment. *American Journal of Occupational Therapy*, **42**(5), 288–95.

Patient's Charter (1991) Department of Health, HMSO, London.

Peloquin, S. (1993) Depersonalisation of patients: a profile gleaned from narratives. *American Journal of Occupational Therapy*, **47**(9), 830–7.

Ryan, S. (1995) Teaching clinical reasoning skills to occupational therapy students during fieldwork education. In J. Higgs and M. Jones (eds), *Clinical Reasoning in the Health Professions*. Butterworth-Heinemann, Oxford, 246–57.

Sacks, O. (1986) *The Man Who Mistook His Wife for a Hat*. Pan Books, London.

Sacks, O. (1995) *An Anthropologist on Mars*. Picador, London.

Schwartzberg, S. (1992) Self-disclosure and empathy in occupational therapy, Paper presented at the Occupational Therapy Conference, Trinity College, Dublin, Ireland, July 1992.

Slater, D. (1989) Developing reflective practitioners in the clinic. Paper presented at the American Occupational Therapy Association Conference, Baltimore MD.

Turner, A., Foster, M. and Johnson, S. (eds) (1992) *Occupational Therapy and Physical Dysfunction*, 3rd edn, Churchill Livingstone, Edinburgh.

Wallis D. and Hutchings, S. (1990) The attainment of professional attitudes; the use of group based work in a clinical and school based setting. *British Journal of Occupational Therapy*. **53**(2), 48–52.

Weimer, R. (1994) *Student transition from academic to fieldwork settings*. In *Guide to Fieldwork Education*, American Occupational Therapy Association, 171-7.

World Health Organization (1980) *International Classification of Impairments, Disabilities and Handicaps*. WHO, Geneva.

The first few days 10

This chapter covers:

- matters relating to your accommodation while on placement;
- the induction programme;
- the first meeting with your fieldwork educator;
- the fieldwork setting as a context for learning;
- learning logs and learning contracts;
- early work with clients.

The first day at your placement may be one of great anticipation, even if this is not your first fieldwork experience. But if you have followed some of the suggestions outlined earlier and are well prepared for the new and different demands to be made of you, you can aim to enjoy the placement. In this chapter we take you through what you might expect of those first few days and consider how you might help yourself to settle in, to learn about what is on offer and to discover how to make the most of opportunities to enhance your learning and experience. We start by mentioning some of the practical issues that have to be addressed, and then continue by examining the nature of the early educational experience.

PRACTICAL ARRANGEMENTS

Settling in to your accommodation

Some of you may be fortunate to be able to travel daily from your home to your placement. For others, it means making arrangements for accommodation close by, in a nurses' home for instance, or in other lodgings in the locality. If you are to have hospital accommodation you will be given instructions by your fieldwork educator about collecting the key and finding your room. We advise you to arrive early and leave plenty of time for finding your way around, especially if you are due to arrive on a Sunday when fewer people are available to assist you. Some students prefer to negotiate a later start to their placement so that they can travel and settle in to their accommodation on a weekday. As you settle in, make sure you take the time to find out where fire alarms, exits and appliances are situated.

Facilities available to you

Hospital accommodation is notably sparse, and in lodgings you may feel isolated. You might wish to take some personal items with you for 'home comfort'. Check whether you can have access to any sports, recreational or leisure facilities. You also need to enquire about catering facilities and restaurants and check opening hours. There may be kitchen facilities available to you but if you intend to self-cater you may need to take cooking utensils.

Sadly, theft from buildings (and from refrigerators) is not uncommon so you should lock everything away in your room when not in use. Make sure you keep your belongings safe and secure. Do not leave your door unlocked and check the situation regarding windows. If you have ground floor accommodation, do not leave windows open while you are out, and consider very carefully the extent to which you might leave windows open while you are asleep. Nurses' homes can attract 'opportunists' so you need to take sensible precautions while you are in a strange environment. Last but not least, do not forget to settle any account for the accommodation before you leave!

INDUCTION AND ADMINISTRATION

Induction

Make sure you are punctual and be ready to slot into any programme that has been prepared for you. Ideally, you will be introduced to some of the team members with whom you will be working, and you will spend some time informally with your fieldwork educator clarifying your learning needs and expectations. In hospital situations where patients must be seen early, for certain activities of daily living for instance, the hospital routine may take priority and discussions with your educator may be postponed until later in the day. You should have an induction programme prepared for you which should indicate where you will be working, and with whom. This will help to orientate you to the service before you explore in more detail how your learning needs can be addressed.

Induction programmes vary tremendously so we can only be very general here about the programme you might have. We have given some details below of the kind of issues which are likely to be addressed, such as an introduction to health and safety, the team, the clients and service administration. We suggest you keep a notebook with you so that you can jot down relevant information. You might also take a diary with you to record appointments and key tasks planned for the days ahead. Sometimes the service keeps a diary for use by students which is handed from one student to another. If there is no such diary, then use your own but you will need to take precautions not to breach confidentiality by noting details of clients which might result in their being identified as you take your diary with you at the end of the placement.

You may find that visits have been arranged for you or that appointments have been made for you to spend time with members of other disciplines. There may be staff meetings to note, or in-service training sessions. Often students are invited to join educational activities which are scheduled for staff but which also seem relevant to students. If you have a placement in a teaching hospital or any hospital where there is a post-graduate medical centre there are often presentations which are open to all staff.

Health and safety

As part of your induction you may be required to have a medical or to complete health check forms. You may even be sent for a chest X-ray. Apart from being in your interests, these health checks are in place to safeguard the service and ensure that no-one is employed who is likely to put themselves or others at risk in the course of their work.

By law each service has to make explicit its health and safety policy so there should be a policy and procedures file available for you to consult. You must be aware of health and safety measures taken by the service. Your ability to 'practise safely' is likely to depend on your awareness of these policies and procedures. They will vary according to the client group. For instance, those for mental health and forensic services are likely to be different from those in a district general hospital. In services for people with learning difficulties or for children or adolescents with behavioural problems there may be special policies and procedures.

Sometimes prior to having a placement with children, 'police checks' may have to be carried out on you. Although a Home Office Circular (HOC101/1988) indicates that this procedure is unnecessary for students, some services insist that the procedure is followed. This is nothing to be alarmed about. There has been considerable publicity in the past about employees acting improperly with children and where children have been placed at risk. Police checks ensure that there is no record of any incident that would indicate that you were an unsuitable person to work with children.

The policies and procedures described above are intended to protect the clients, staff and visitors from unnecessary risk or harm and they are extremely important. Additionally, in some services such as secure units, there will be restrictions on movement. Keys may have to be issued, alarm systems and security procedures may have to be explained, and it is essential that you listen and take careful note of what you are told and what you are required to do.

You should certainly familiarize yourself with the fire alarm system and evacuation routes, appliances and procedures. You will also need to know how equipment is stored and secured, and the procedures for dealing with spillages, including spillages of blood or other bodily fluids. Remember, the Health and Safety at Work Act 1974, and its subsequent amendments, apply to you as an individual, a visitor and an employee. Ignorance of the law is no defence when it comes to explaining any actions taken. Although your fieldwork educator will, no doubt, take these responsibilities seriously and induct you as to the various procedures, you too share that responsibility and must ask about the interpretation of health and safety regulations in the local environment.

When you are eager to start your work with clients, familiarizing yourself with health and safety requirements first can seem very mundane. Policies and procedures are there to protect you so you should not dismiss their relevance or importance. You would be exposed to exactly the same induction if you were to be starting a new job.

The environment

Hospitals and other large organizations can seem formidable places and time is needed to get to know them. Your fieldwork educator may take you on a tour of the building or may provide you with a check list of places to locate which will help you to find your bearings. Your mental map of where offices and departments are in relation to each other will soon fall into place. Your fieldwork educator will also tell you about any special procedures for accessing departments such as intensive treatment units or secure environments if your work is likely to entail visits to such places.

The team

Members of the team with whom you will be working will be as keen to meet you as you will be to meet them. After all, for the next few weeks you will be interacting with them and learning from them, so forming and maintaining good working relationships is crucial. Team or group dynamics can so easily be upset by a new member so it is important at any time, and especially during the induction, to be very careful about how you present yourself to the team. Be natural with them, be pleasant and above all be respectful of them, and of their role and experience. You may find yourselves working alongside support workers or Occupational Therapy assistants. These people often have very special skills, and sometimes technical skills, and they play a very important role in the delivery of service to clients. Sometimes it can be difficult for Occupational Therapy students to know what kind of relationship it is appropriate for them to have with these members of staff. It is worth remembering that every member of the team, regardless of grade or qualification makes a unique contribution to the team and your relationship with each one of them will be as a colleague.

Administration

Administration systems will vary from service to service, but as a minimum you will need to find out how the telephone system works, what arrangements there are for recording messages and what system is in use for determining staff movements and for knowing who is in or out of the building.

Other administrative systems relate more to service provision and the indirect care activities undertaken by therapists, support workers and administrative staff. Although you may be introduced to some of these systems as part of your induction you will almost certainly learn about other systems as you need to use them. They include:

- the referral system;
- the duty system;
- the system for booking transport;
- the system for arranging porters;
- the system for issuing equipment;
- the system for completing sales, issuing receipts and handling cash;
- the system for recording interventions ie.writing client notes;
- the system for recording data about clients, their attendances and their contacts with staff for statistical purposes.

Some of these systems may be computerized and you will need to learn how to access and input data.

Again this is not an all-inclusive list and you will find many other systems in use in the services you visit. In those services which have their policies and procedures files up to date you should find an explanation of how the systems work and examples of the forms used. You will also need to remember that systems change very frequently and keeping these files up-to-date is a very arduous task, and one often neglected. The one thing that might strike you, however, is just how much administrative work is involved in the process of care delivery, and how time-consuming it is to complete. Almost without exception you will find occupational therapists complaining about the high proportion of their time spent completing administrative tasks. Unfortunately this is increasing because of the purchaser/provider arrangements and the need for accurate information to inform the service costing process. It is not unusual for occupational therapists to bemoan the fact that they entered the profession so that they could work closely with people, yet the administration of care delivery so often keeps them away from their clients.

Client records

One of the most time consuming tasks for occupational therapists is writing client records, but equally it is one of the most important tasks which supports care delivery. In brief, client records are important legal documents which serve as a reference for therapists and team members and which reflect their activity with clients. You will know from your academic studies that client records:

- provide baseline information collected from interviews, assessments, interactions and interventions with clients on which care plans are formulated and monitored;

- indicate the plan of action negotiated and agreed between client and therapist;
- specify action taken to date, client responses, outcomes of interventions and problems which remain unresolved.

Client records should be legible, complete, concise, accurate, up-to-date, and signed and dated by the writer. They should be written, consulted and kept confidential in accordance with the policies and conventions of the service.

There are many record systems in existence, each with its own structure and format, so it is impossible for you to know them all. You should therefore expect your fieldwork educator to explain the one in use in that service.

Structures for record-keeping can be multi-disciplinary or profession-specific. Sometimes records are kept separately by individual professions and readily accessible by members of that profession alone, and sometimes there is a central record-keeping system which is consulted and used by all members of the multi-disciplinary team. Often nurses have their own systems. If you are allowed to access them for information about clients you will need to understand their structure and format and where relevant information may be found. Occupational therapists often use a format for client records which reflects the model or approach used for client care. For instance, the format of records may be based on the Model of Human Occupation (Kielhofner, 1985) or the Reed and Sanderson Process Model (1983). Individual professions or multi-disciplinary teams may use a more universal structure such as that of Problem Oriented Medical Records (POMR) (Weed, 1971).

For each placement you should clarify the system of record-keeping used. You should also ask specifically how you should sign the records and whether your fieldwork educator needs to countersign them. You have to remember that as a consequence of the Access to Health Records Act 1990 and the equivalent local authority regulations – Access to Personal Files (Social Services) (Amendment) Regulations 1991, clients can seek access to their records by following the appropriate procedure. Apart from being good practice, this is one of the reasons that you should take extreme care about what you write about clients and how you write it. No tippex or whitener should ever be used in client records and anything you do write should be based on fact and be presented in an objective and professional way. There is always the chance, however slight, that a client's records may be used as a basis of evidence in a court of law and scrutinized by the judge should a client ever take legal action relating to services received. As a technical instructor in an Occupational Therapy service, Rob Bryant (1993) recorded his experience of having reports he had written submitted to defence solicitors as part of a court action. The prospect of becoming a witness caused him anxiety, even though the case was ultimately settled out of court.

Abbreviations

One other thing that you must be sure about is the meaning of abbreviations used at your placement. Each service will use a set of abbreviations for both verbal and written communication which is peculiar to that service. You must ensure that you understand these abbreviations and do not jump to conclusions about their meaning based on your experience at other placements or places of employment. Often fieldwork educators prepare a list of commonly used abbreviations and their meanings as a handout and this can be most useful as a reference. If there is no list, then we recommend that you make one for yourself as you come across the terms and then leave a copy for the department.

Other practical matters

Before the first official meeting with your educator it might be useful for you to make a note of any issues that you would like to raise. Time will almost certainly be short, and a list will help you to address any essential areas of concern. Some of the more practical points you might discuss are as follows:

- health-related matters which might affect the placement;
- limitations in your knowledge and experience in relation to the tasks you may be asked to perform eg. lifting and handling clients;
- to whom you should turn for support and guidance in the absence of your fieldwork educator;
- how you should claim travel expenses incurred on placement, and expectations and limitations of your role if expenses cannot be claimed.

You also need to clarify the following issues which relate to your education on placement:

- expectations of the fieldwork educator regarding written work;
- academic work required by the university;
- time off for study leave.

Table 10.1 summarizes the items which might be included in an induction programme.

Table 10.1 Induction guidelines

- Introductions
- Working site arrangements
- Orientation to the service
- Medical check-up/X-ray
- Health and safety policy and procedures
- Fire alarm systems
- Location of store for equipment
- Finding your way around (checklist and map)
- Find out about the telephone system for clients' notes
- Abbreviations used

EDUCATIONAL NEEDS, STRATEGIES AND OPPORTUNITIES

The first meeting with your fieldwork educator

The primary purpose of the first meeting with your fieldwork educator is to gain an understanding of the placement as a context for learning, and to clarify:

- the learning opportunities available;
- your learning needs and goals;
- your responsibilities with clients;
- the arrangements for your supervision.

The outcome of the first meeting with your fieldwork educator should be an agreement about your contribution to client care for the first few days of the placement and the learning goals to be achieved during this time. The date and time for reflecting upon, and evaluating these experiences through supervision should be known.

Keeping a learning log or diary

The main reason for you being at the placement is to learn about clients, their needs and their care management, and to explore how occupational therapists contribute to that process within the wider context of the organization. The placement provides you with the context of learning, but it is from your own experiences in that setting that most of your learning will occur. Much of your learning will come from the process of reflection which we discuss more fully in Chapter 15. Here we want to recommend that you record your learning experiences as part of that reflective process.

Keeping a learning log or diary is one way of recording your experiences, your reactions, your feelings, your thoughts and your observations. These observations will stem from your interactions with clients and their carers, from those engaged in care delivery and from many other sources such as meetings, interventions, visits, literature and from informal conversation. These are the triggers of learning; but the quality of your learning will be enhanced if you think through and record the issues which emerge. Sarah Beeston (personal communication, September 1995) explains the difference between a log and a diary. She suggests that a log records events and tracks progress whereas a diary contains personal interpretations of events. Feelings as well as facts can be recorded. A journal, on the other hand, is a blend of the two. It can contain structured, descriptive notes as well as the free-flowing meanderings of a diary.

Honey and Mumford (1992) suggest that learning should not be left to chance and that it is best done as a deliberate, conscious process as a learning log. They believe that the log should contain a record of the event but also of the learning that derived from it. Determining the information entails:

- thinking back over the experience and selecting a part of it that was significant or important to you;
- writing a detailed account of what happened (without saying what you learned);

- listing the conclusions reached as a result of the experience (these are your learning points);
- deciding how you are going to use the learning which has occurred.

This is a good structure to use as a starting point for recording your learning experience. As you get used to evaluating your experiences your writing may become more sophisticated. You may think that you have learned something from an experience without needing to write it down. This is probably so. The process of recording your experiences is about enhancing your learning and making sure that you do gain the most from reflecting on the opportunities you have had.

The service context, philosophy and approach to work

The placement is the context in which you will gain your fieldwork experience, but what you learn and how you learn will depend on the service philosophy, the resources available and the way in which they are used. There is much to learn from the wider organization in which you work, and we will return to this point shortly. The Occupational Therapy service, however, is likely to be part of a wider service and the profession's activity will be underpinned by the philosophy and mission statement adopted by the service as a whole.

The service philosophy and mission statement therefore guide the work of the organization and its staff. You may already have an indication of the philosophy from the briefing pack sent to you prior to the placement. This is the time to clarify your understanding of it, and the way it influences the work undertaken by practitioners with their clients. In some services all practitioners in the multi-disciplinary team use a common approach, in other services practitioners use a profession-specific approach which is compatible with the wider service philosophy.

Some practitioners adopt one clear model for practice, such as the Model of Human Occupation (Kielhofner, 1985), the Model of Personal Adaptation (Reed and Sanderson, 1983), the Sensory Integrative Approach (Ayres, 1972) or the Canadian Occupational Performance Measure (Law *et al.*, 1994). Other practitioners adopt a more eclectic approach drawing on a range of theoretical frameworks as necessary, e.g. the biomechanical, developmental and/or rehabilitative framework to guide their work. In order to understand the language and terms used by members of the team it is important for you to ascertain this information very early on, otherwise you will find it difficult to communicate with staff about clients and to collaborate with the team to provide client care in an informed way. You obviously need to adopt the same approach for your work and to be able to use the principles of the preferred theoretical approach confidently in your practice.

Learning opportunities and resources

Learning opportunities will be found largely within the organization, from experiences with clients and those involved in delivering client care. Many more opportunities for learning may be available to you than you can possibly hope to take advantage of, and some careful selection may need to take place. It may be suggested that you go on visits or spend time in other services or with other professionals. Many of these experiences will be invaluable but you may have to be selective. Clearly you need to consider your previous experience, your present level of professional development and your identified learning needs. You may need to discriminate between useful and less useful learning opportunities at that time.

Most learning will come from your interaction with people, but there are other resources which should be available to support your learning. You need to find out whether there is a library, whether you have any other access to books, whether you can borrow them or only use them for reference within the department, and whether you may use a photocopier. You need to know whether there is a quiet room where you can read and write notes as part of your studies. Some services are geared to students and can readily identify facilities for learning, others are so lacking in space that a room for educational studies is just not available. Other arrangements will then need to be negotiated. You will need to clarify what resources you have access to, and how they may be used.

Your learning needs and goals

The learning contract and placement objectives

Tomkins and McGraw (1988) state that a learning contract is a continuously negotiable working agreement between student and teacher which emphasizes mutuality in decision-making and student self-determination in relation to learning outcomes. The aim of a learning contract is really to make explicit the expectations that the educator has of you, and that you have of yourself and your educator, in relation to meeting your learning needs. The most important factor, however, is that of continuous negotiation to ensure that the learning contract changes to meet changing needs, rather than serving as a single contract which is in place from the beginning to the end of the placement.

Any contract is an agreement between two parties with an expectation that the conditions specified within it will be met by the parties concerned. There are normally several stages to the learning contract as follows.

1. clarification of current knowledge and skills;
2. identification of learning needs;
3. exploration of learning opportunities available;
4. specification of goals and learning outcomes;
5. formulation of a plan of action;
6. division of responsibilities between the parties concerned;
7. determination of a time scale for achieving goals and outcomes;
8. evaluation of outcomes against established goals;
9. re-negotiation of contract to reflect future learning needs.

The goals, outcomes, action plan and responsibilities are set down in writing as a contract and as a reference for determining whether goals have been achieved. The criteria against which outcomes will be measured are made explicit to avoid any subsequent misunderstandings.

Where you are required to negotiate and work to a learning contract you will need to consider very carefully the degree to which the desired outcomes are achievable in the time available to you, and with the resources accessible to you. You will also need to consider the terms of the contract in relation to your placement, including its aims and objectives and the learning outcomes on which you will be assessed. The learning contract needs to be consistent with the requirements of your educational programme and its objectives. It also must take account of your current level of professional development, an area often neglected by fieldwork educators whose expectations of students can sometimes be unrealistically high.

Where you are not working to the formality of a learning contract you will still have placement objectives. These are usually determined by your fieldwork educator, in consultation with yourself. The fieldwork educator will adapt the objectives set by the university to produce locally relevant objectives which indicate what you will be required to do in that service to meet the placement requirements. Your contract and/or the extent to which you are achieving your learning objectives should be reviewed regularly, usually weekly, with your fieldwork educator and any adjustments made to your programme at the time.

Your responsibilities with clients

When you meet your fieldwork educator for your first discussion you should be given details of your programme and an opportunity to clarify expectations and to negotiate any changes needed. You should also receive details of the clients with whom you will be expected to work and be guided as to how to approach your responsibilities with them. Even at this early stage of the placement the fieldwork educator may test out your knowledge of clinical conditions by asking you how you might proceed with such clients, and about the characteristics of the condition which need to be taken into consideration in the care management process. If you have done your preparatory reading you should be able to answer such questions quite freely, and you should be well enough prepared to be able to ask informed questions at the briefing session about clients and their problems. Beware, however, a good fieldwork educator may not necessarily provide you with a straightforward answer to your questions but suggest the means whereby you might find out for yourself!

Meeting the clients

Arrangements should be made for you to meet clients very early in your placement, preferably on the first day. Much will depend on the type of service in which you are gaining your experience and whether clients are readily accessible. For instance, in a hospital situation, inpatients are likely to be accessible because they are receiving treatment there, but for community services you may be based in a team office and need to go out to various home addresses in order to meet clients. This may or may not be done through an appointment system. Day patients and outpatients will attend a service according to their schedule and you will meet them at that time.

On your first placement in a community setting you will almost certainly accompany your fieldwork educator on his or her visits to clients in the first instance. You should have an opportunity to observe clients and carers and their interactions with your educator, and you may have a chance to participate in the discussions. While observing the interactions you should note the approach that your educator takes with the clients, and their responses. Ideally, after each visit to a client you should have an opportunity to reflect on your observations and to discuss the therapeutic encounter. This will be a first step to you gaining the confidence and experience necessary to take the lead on visits to other clients.

Over the first couple of weeks in your placement, the natural progression would be for you first to observe, then participate in, and finally lead discussions under supervision, before carrying out visits alone and reporting back to your fieldwork educator. It is unlikely that you would be asked to visit clients alone until you had gained the relevant experience and confidence by working with your educator on several visits.

On your first placement, meeting clients on wards of a district general hospital would probably follow the same pattern. You would accompany your fieldwork educator, observe the assessments and interactions and then participate in treatment regimes as directed until you had the confidence to undertake assessments and treatment sessions alone and report back. Don't forget that the process of reflection on your practice at this early stage of your experience is crucial to your learning and professional development.

Your first meeting with clients being treated in mental health services or services for people with learning difficulties may be somewhat different. If you have never been in contact with clients with these kinds of problems, and you have reservations about how to approach them, then do speak to your fieldwork educator about your concerns. It is far better to be honest and to seek some help in preparing for what is to come. For instance, there may be videos which you could watch first and then discuss with your fieldwork educator to help you work through some of your anxieties.

Your fieldwork educator should guide you as to the approach to take and may give you some hints on behaviour to avoid. Your educator will know the clients individually and will have an understanding of their problems and needs. He or she should enable you to start interacting with clients in a safe and sensible manner so that you can begin to feel comfortable about working with them. It may take you a while to get used to certain kinds of behaviour. Use supervision sessions to discuss your feelings and your progress in adapting to the circumstances of the placement.

Your relationship with clients

Clients may be interested in the fact that you are a student but they will expect you to act as a professional and behave as a trainee practitioner. You will have to put your student status to one side and perform as a professional at all times. Essentially this means putting clients and their needs before your own. You need to be able to share a conversation with clients, to listen carefully to what they say, to work with them to help them determine **their** needs, to seek out **their** expectations and to find out **their** concerns and hopes for the future. You may not be able to answer their questions, in fact it is preferable for you to leave sensitive issues to those qualified to discuss them, but you can aim to put clients at their ease and to be honest about your position as a trainee. You would be well advised to focus on clients' problems and future needs rather than on their diagnosis, which they may not know. You will need to avoid making suggestions or promises which you might be unable to fulfil. You should keep the conversation informal, but still professional. The conversation need not be serious, nor without laughter, but you should take great care about how you use humour as it can so easily be misconstrued and offend. Remember, clients are in a very vulnerable position and often more sensitive to their situation than is immediately apparent.

Your socialization into the wider organization

Your fieldwork experience is a time when you can expect to be oriented to the way in which the profession operates, and to the language and the culture of the profession, that is your **professional socialization**. There is another form of socialization, however, that of **organizational socialization** which will start to take place as you participate in the activities of the service. This is quite an important aspect of your learning, and again not overtly addressed in the literature about fieldwork education.

As a temporary employee in an organization, you will begin to learn how the organization operates, what influences its operations, where and how the profession makes its contribution and how individual members perform their role. You will gain insights into the demands of the worker role and an awareness of the reality and pressures of work. You will be exposed to a range of organizational behaviours where individuals pursue personal interests and goals in the process of delivering services to clients. These experiences of organizational life are just as valid and important as the professional experience you gain in Occupational Therapy. They contribute significantly to your preparation for professional life.

As part of the learning process you should take opportunities to explore the effectiveness of service provision and the way in which the organization meets its goals through the efforts of its employees. You might evaluate the influences on the organization of external factors such as social policy, and the relationship of the organization with other agencies; you might examine internal factors such as organizational policies and management structures and their effects on service delivery. These are all part of the service context and the setting for your learning experience. The quality of service provided to clients by occupational therapists is likely to be influenced quite strongly by many of these factors. You should therefore not underestimate the extent to which knowledge of the organization and the way it functions can help you in your understanding of Occupational Therapy practice.

The first week

By the end of the first week much of what is on offer at the placement should be apparent to you. You will have begun to identify the key members of staff who will enable your learning, you will have some idea of what the organization has to offer, and you will have gained some appreciation of what you can learn from clients and your interactions with them. Do not underestimate the extent to which each of these three resources (staff, organization and clients) can assist your educational and professional development. Make sure that you examine issues relating to service delivery and intervention programmes from all three perspectives as information gained from only one source is unlikely to present you with the whole picture of client care management.

If you consider service delivery in its widest sense, and from all three perspectives, it should help you to learn to research, evaluate and present a balanced discussion on the issues concerned – all important skills for professional life. Your placement resembles the work situation when you qualify and you will draw on the same three sources of information in employment as an occupational therapist.

You will almost certainly find that the first week goes very quickly and at the end of it you will be very tired. As we have shown, there is a good deal to learn in a new environment and you are expected to adjust to the new situation very quickly. It is important that you do adjust, because you are a temporary member of staff and you cannot expect other people to change what they do just because of your presence. You are the one who will have to fit in, if you do not, this may cause tension which can be disruptive to client care. If there are circumstances in which you feel uncomfortable or do not understand, then you should raise the issues with your fieldwork educator as soon as practicable. Do ensure, however, that matters of concern are discussed in private and not in public.

SUMMARY

This chapter has addressed issues relevant to your entry into the placement and your induction to the policies, systems and resources which will support your practice and facilitate your studies. In particular, Health and Safety policies and client record systems have been discussed. The chapter has introduced you to some strategies for learning, such as keeping a learning log and formulating a learning contract, and for making the most of the opportunities available to you. Strategies for taking responsibility for clients' care management and for assuming a role in the wider organization have also been examined.

REFERENCES

Ayers, A. J. (1972) *Sensory Integration and Learning Disorders,* Western Psychological Services, Los Angeles.

Bryant, R (1993) Doing Justice to the OT Client. *Therapy Weekly*, **19**(40), 22 April 1993.

Honey, P. and Mumford, A. (1992) *The Manual of Learning Styles*, 3rd edn. Peter Honey, Ardingley House, Linden Ave., Maidenhead, Berks. England.

Kielhofner, G. (1995) *A Model of Human Occupation: Theory and Application*, 2nd edn. Williams & Wilkins, Baltimore.

Law, M., Baptiste, S., Carswell, A., McColl, M. A., Polatajko, H. and Pollock, N. (1994) *Canadian Occupational Performance Measure Manual*, 2nd edn. Canadian Occupational Therapy Publications, Toronto.

Reed, K. L and Sanderson, S. R. (1983) *Concepts of Occupational Therapy*, 2nd edn. Williams & Wilkins, Baltimore.

Tomkins, C. and McGraw, M. J. (1988) The *Negotiated Student Contract*. In Boud, D. (ed.), *Developing Student Autonomy in Learning*, 2nd edn. Kogan Page, London.

Weed, L. L. (1971) *Medical Records, Medical Educations and Patient Care*. Case Western Reserve University Press, Cleveland, OH.

11 Participating in service delivery

This chapter covers:

- an overview of the organization as a context for fieldwork;
- making a contribution to the care of clients through teamwork;
- learning from occupational therapists, clients and other professionals;
- practising without discrimination.

As you settle in to the fieldwork setting you will begin to appreciate the contribution that you can make to client care through participating in service delivery. You will be part of a team within the wider organization, collaborating with colleagues from different professions but drawing on Occupational Therapy approaches, processes and skills to bring a unique professional dimension to the management of client care. In many ways, the contribution that you make will draw as much on your personal qualities and skills as on those professional skills and qualities that you are developing as an occupational therapist. You will thus find that fieldwork will help you to develop and grow both personally and professionally as you face and meet the challenges of this part of your educational programme.

In order to make a contribution to service delivery you will need to develop an understanding of the organizational structure in which you are working and adapt to it fairly quickly. You will need to learn to operate in accordance with the organizational philosophy and to work with the team in an effective way. You will also need to recognize the strengths and limitations of the service in which you are working and to be able to appreciate the extent to which it can, and does, meet client needs. Your participation in service delivery depends on you being able to fit into the environment and take responsibility for selected aspects of client care according to your level of knowledge and experience.

UNDERSTANDING THE ORGANIZATION

We mentioned earlier in the book that the organizational context in which your fieldwork experience takes place is an important learning environment. This is the environment in which clients receive their care, the environment in which your needs take second place to their needs. However, as the context of providing for the needs of clients, the organization becomes one of the most effective learning environments that you can possibly have. The more that you can learn about the service and how it meets its goals, the greater will be your understanding of the role which occupational therapists play in service delivery.

The influence of social policy

One of the biggest influences on the service is legislation, which not only guides the service philosophy but also its organizational and management structure. The National Health Service and Community Care Act 1990 is currently one of the most influential pieces of legislation on health and social care provision. This Act gave impetus to community care, created the purchaser/provider arrangements and established self-governing NHS Trusts. Other legislation provides the legal frameworks within which occupational therapists work, depending on the employing authority and client group served. Some of the relevant Acts of Parliament are listed in Appendix B. From legislation comes the service philosophy, the beliefs which guide the manner in which services are delivered.

The organizational philosophy

The organizational philosophy and any mission statement adopted, reflect the operations of the total service, which includes Occupational Therapy. Teams often have their own mission statement, as do many Occupational Therapy services. This indicates the preferred approach to meeting client needs. A philosophy adopted by the Occupational Therapy profession normally takes account, not only of the physical and psychological manifestations of a client's condition which interfere with his or her ability to be productive in society, but also of the social context and environment in which a client chooses to function, and the individual's capacity to adapt to changing needs and circumstances within his or her life, and life roles.

Dilemmas in service delivery

As a student, you may come face to face with all sorts of dilemmas relating to service delivery, some of which may seem very uncomfortable. Many facets of organizational life bring pressures and challenges for occupational therapists as providers of services and often result in hard decisions having to be made. In order for you to come to terms with choices and priorities in service delivery, you need to consider the effects of social policy and the context in which services are delivered. An awareness of the issues should give you some insight into the difficult choices which have to be made and the various dimensions and perspectives which have to be taken into consideration in making those choices. Ask questions of team members to clarify issues which arise. The more widely you think about service provision for the total population which the organization serves (rather than just about the specific interventions for individual clients) the better your appreciation of the problems and ethical dilemmas which care providers must face and resolve. Some ethical problems encountered by therapists are addressed in an article by Barnitt (1993) which we would recommend to students embarking on fieldwork.

The organizational structure

Every organization has its own structure through which it delivers its services. The structure provides the management framework and determines how the service is divided functionally, demographically or geographically in order to meet its responsibilities to clients and fulfil its goals. The organization will almost certainly be divided up into smaller **units** or teams which will have responsibility for discrete aspects of client care. In collaboration with other teams, each will contribute to the total work of the wider organization.

Teams within the organization

On placement you could find yourself working both in a profession-specific team offering Occupational Therapy services to clients, and in a multi-disciplinary team which provides more comprehensive services and which draws on a variety of skills to meet client needs. The multi-disciplinary team may operate in one of several different ways, for instance:

- geographically in a locality, patch or neighbourhood serving the needs of all clients in the area;
- demographically as a clinical directorate or team providing specialist services for a specific age-related population, for instance, children, adults, or elderly people; or
- functionally serving clients with particular problems, for instance mental health problems, physical disability, learning difficulties.

The expertise and skill mix within the team will depend on the way in which services are organized and the relationships which exist between different services and other local agencies.

Within the literature and in practice, you will find reference to the terms multi-disciplinary, inter-disciplinary and trans-disciplinary. These terms refer to the different ways in which teams of health professionals work together.

Multi-disciplinary refers to a team of health professionals who come together with their different professional skills. Each person provides a unique perspective on what needs to be done. A decision is then taken on the way to proceed. Each person thus makes a discrete contribution to the team through the way that he or she thinks and acts.

Inter-disciplinary refers to a team of health professionals who know each other well, who acknowledge their overlapping professional skills and decide together who will do whatever is needed. For example, several team members might have foundation counselling skills but one member has a better personal rapport with the client. The team decides that that person will counsel the client. As with the multidisciplinary team, each professional still contributes his or her own specific skills.

Trans-disciplinary refers to a team of people who have all agreed to work in a particular way and each person contributes towards the overall care of clients. Each person is trained to perform the skills necessary for providing the programme, so knowledge and skills are generic. This way of working is particularly appropriate for places providing in-house services like those in elderly care facilities and short-term treatment centres.

By examining Figure 11.1 carefully, you can see that the relationships between the members will be quite different depending on the way in which the team is working. Being alert to the differences will help you to understand the function, dynamics and effectiveness of team approaches to care management.

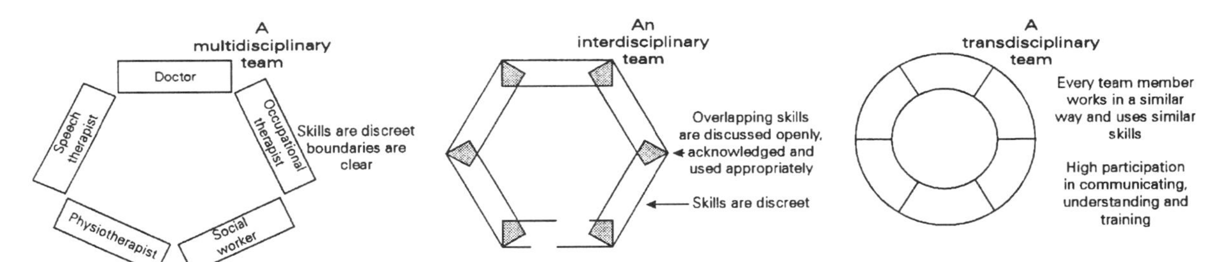

Figure 11.1 Different team configurations

THE MANAGEMENT OF THE ORGANIZATION

Each team is likely to be headed by a service manager. This person may be someone who has a background in one of the caring professions but who has moved into a management role, or an individual who has trained exclusively in the field of management but who has little, or no, hands-on experience of care delivery with clients. Clinical directorates may be headed by a consultant or by a professional who undertakes a joint management/clinical role. Whoever heads up a service will be responsible and accountable for the resources allocated to it, and for the activity of the team.

One thing to remember about participating in service delivery is that occupational therapists are rarely service managers who have total control over Occupational Therapy resources, or the way in which they are deployed. Decisions about resource allocation and about service delivery are more likely to be made by an executive board or committee, or by an individual who has limited knowledge of Occupational Therapy. An awareness of the decision making processes will often help explain any mismatch between the profession's desire to provide an effective Occupational Therapy service to a given client group, and the more limited service which is actually provided in practice. It may also help to explain any discrepancy between the theory you have learned in the university, and what you see taking place within the service.

If you feel uncomfortable about the level of Occupational Therapy service provided to clients, you can be sure that these same sentiments are shared by many members of the profession. The restrictions on service delivery, which often result from resource constraints, deny occupational therapists the opportunity to work autonomously and to use their wide-ranging skills to meet clients' total functional needs. The outcome for the clients receiving these services may be an improved ability to perform activities of daily living safely, but clients may never achieve the level of independence of which they are capable and which they desire. It is for these reasons that therapists need to adapt service delivery, advocate needs and carry out research to illustrate efficiency and effectiveness of their programmes of intervention.

Of course there will always be constraints. As part of the reality of service provision you will almost certainly be exposed to the way in which the profession determines its priorities, the dilemmas of waiting lists and the difficulties arising from resource constraints (Scrivens, 1982). If you stop for a moment and analyse the outside influences on the organization, the internal organizational structure and management arrangements for the service, these may help to explain how resources and services are balanced for efficiency and effectiveness. It is really important, therefore, that you do not lose sight of the strengths of the service, the outcomes for clients and the standards that are achieved in the delivery of client care, i.e. the positive aspects of care delivery and not just the limitations. Your fieldwork educator should be able to help you think through these issues and so enhance your understanding of organizational life and of the services provided to clients.

Communicating with the team

Effective service delivery depends essentially on the quality of communication between all those involved in client care. Good working relationships, networks, structures and systems, and consistency in approach are vital. Smaller units provide the team structure and will certainly be the primary focus of communication. We have already mentioned team dynamics and the importance of interpersonal relationships within the team. Just stop and think for a moment of all the factors which might contribute to **ineffective** teamwork, and their consequences. You may be quite surprised to discover just how many factors are involved in maintaining effective communication and how quickly communication can break down. If you think these through, you should then begin to appreciate the part that you will need to play in maintaining adequate standards of client care through appropriate communication with members of the team.

There are different media for communicating. Figure 11.2 illustrates various channels of communication that can be used in health and social care. Although you may have a preferred medium, it is worth finding out what others use in their particular setting. You may have ideas about improving channels of communication which you can put to your fieldwork educator for discussion.

FINDING YOUR FEET

Your induction programme should have provided you with the essential details of the service. In the early stages of your placement you will spend some time with

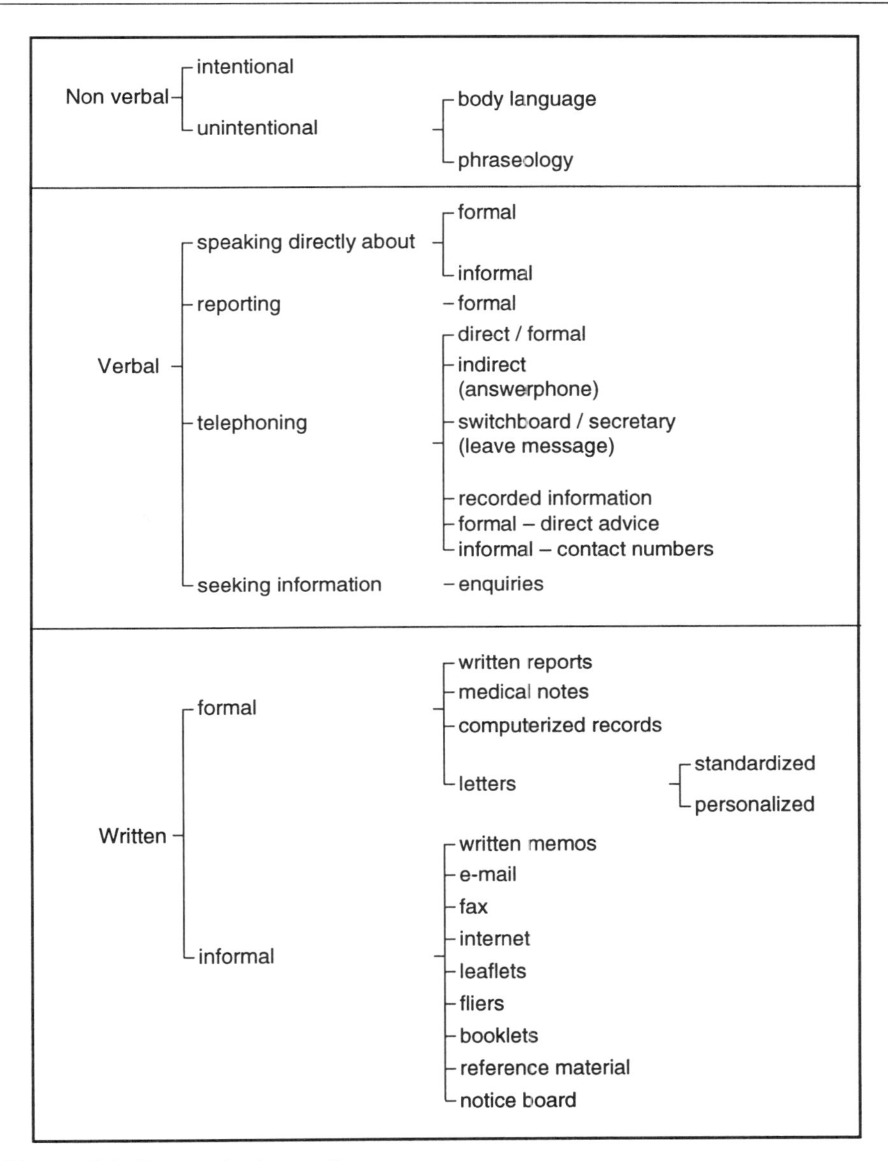

Figure 11.2 Communication media

your fieldwork educator familiarizing yourself with client needs and the approach used to address those needs. There will come a time, however, when you will be given responsibility for a case, and later a caseload, which you must manage for yourself. However daunting this may seem, always remember that you are working under supervision of a qualified practitioner and any action you plan or undertake with the client should normally be discussed first, and also afterwards in a debriefing session.

As you find your feet and participate in service delivery you will be expected to take some initiative and some decisions alone. You will find that responsibility will increase with your level of professional development and your progress through the course. You will ultimately have to demonstrate that you can make an effective contribution to client care through your own efforts and so prove your competence to practise.

You will almost certainly find that the team members with whom you work will be helpful and constructive, and will encourage you to participate in the decisions of the team. You can help yourself by being very clear about the client's needs, about your contribution to the client's care and about the client's response to intervention. The process of reflection will help you to explore those activities in which you have participated, and to explain their consequences. You should be well prepared for any team meeting where a client's needs are discussed, and if you have worked with the client, be ready to contribute to the discussion and to justify any comments you make. Prepare notes before the event to assist you, make sure that you have access to any records of the client's assessment and intervention so that you can refer to them, and be accurate in the information that you are contributing. If other members of the Occupational Therapy team have contributed to the client's care, be sure to seek their comments beforehand, especially if you have to represent them at a meeting.

MANAGING A CASE

It has been said (Christie *et al.*, 1985) that students like to have hands-on experience of providing client care early in their placement. Opportunities for observation, which often precede hands-on opportunities, serve their purpose but do not replace the experience gained from active involvement with clients. You will need to agree with your educator the responsibilities that you can take at different stages of your placement. This is likely to depend on your stage of professional development and on the specialist nature of the service.

In order to assume some responsibility for a client's care you will need to be clear about how the principles of Occupational Therapy are applied in the service in which you are working. A good basic knowledge of the Occupational Therapy process, such as that propounded by Reed and Sanderson (1993) often provides a framework for managing client care. The different stages of the process: referral, assessment or evaluation of need, planning, intervention, evaluation of results and communication with others, provide reference points in the progress of a client's management programme. This problem-solving process model provides the security of a structure and allows work to progress sequentially and in a meaningful way. It has to be said, however, that the problem-solving process model has its critics.

There are those who argue that such a structure can prove rigid and can inhibit the creative thinking for which occupational therapists are renowned. It is also said that the model does not allow for all the unexpected eventualities that inevitably occur as a result of clients' responses to their programme. While the process model provides a safe structure, it also creates a less flexible structure for acknowledging and responding to the different needs of clients. You therefore need to be alert to the potential consequences of pursuing a more systematic approach to problem-solving. An alternative spiral model which acknowledges uncertainties is presented for consideration in Chapter 14 as we suggest how your reasoning skills can develop.

Early in your fieldwork experience, you would normally be given responsibility for selected aspects of client care, working under supervision. Before the end of a first placement you would expect to take responsibility for one or two clients at a time, and possibly more, depending on the circumstances. Taking responsibility for a case may or may not allow you to work through all the stages of the problem-solving process described above. In acute services, problem identification and problem resolution have to be managed very quickly, almost spontaneously, because of service pressures for discharging clients. Conversely, in services for people with learning difficulties or long-term mental health problems, small changes in an individual's functional ability may take a considerable time to achieve.

Carrying a caseload

As you progress in your course and gain experience through fieldwork you will be expected to take responsibility for managing a small caseload of clients who have a variety of problems. In doing this, you will begin to identify with the reality of work and the pressures which occupational therapists experience. You will deal with a number of fairly complex cases simultaneously and must find a way of addressing the differing needs of clients who are at different stages of a rehabilitation programme, both efficiently and effectively. You will find that caseload management becomes a juggling act within the time available and that your ability to seek out and process relevant information, prioritize and solve problems has to keep pace with service demands.

You can see that, for you to do this effectively, it is essential that you prepare well for the placement by reading around the conditions that you might expect to see and by revising relevant knowledge, for instance anatomy, so that you have this at your fingertips when it is required.

Contributing to therapeutic intervention

As a student you will contribute to the care of a number of clients during your fieldwork experience. Because of the range of settings in which you might be based it is impossible in this book to offer guidance about specific Occupational Therapy intervention with clients with whom you might work. Other specialized texts should be consulted for this purpose. In this book we offer you the principles of how you might approach fieldwork, and therapeutic intervention, in any situation.

Wherever you are on placement, one of the aims will be for you to increase your awareness of therapeutic skills and media in use with the clients. You will need to learn how to analyse, select, use and modify media for therapeutic intervention, and how to evaluate the effects of your intervention with clients. By observing, participating in, and reflecting upon therapeutic activity in which occupational therapists engage, you will build up your repertoire of skills and develop your ability to practise as an occupational therapist. We have stressed the relevance and importance of developing these skills throughout the book. You can see here how they are put to constructive use as tools for learning.

In the fieldwork setting you will be practising under supervision in a relatively safe environment. With the agreement of your educator you may be able to experiment with particular therapeutic interventions and try out your own ideas. You will, of course, need to be very clear about the aims or goals of the intervention you propose and you must be able to justify your chosen therapeutic activity and subsequently to be able to evaluate the effectiveness of your intervention.

A recent study on clinical reasoning development (Robertson, 1995) has indicated that in order to obtain optimal results with clients, the fieldwork educator should assist the inexperienced student to formulate the problems to be addressed and identify a variety of solutions. The student should then work out the different processes that might be used to resolve problems and achieve the desired goals. This provides the student with an incomplete framework to guide his or her thinking, but does not provide prescriptive solutions to the problems identified. Plans should then be discussed with the fieldwork educator and the most appropriate path chosen for the client. Robertson's recommendations are fairly new so fieldwork educators may not yet be aware of this strategy for developing your skills. You may need to suggest the exercise to your fieldwork educator and practise it together.

Threats to your safety and violence at work

This section is not intended to alarm you about practice but to advise you in a practical way about potential hazards as you carry out your work. After all, 'forewarned is forearmed'. The nature of occupational therapists' work means that they are very likely to work in statutory or voluntary organizations with clients who potentially may demonstrate unpredictable, threatening or violent behaviour. Incidents may occur either in hospital settings or in the community so occupational therapists need to be aware of policies and procedures for dealing with situations where they feel that their safety may be at risk.

The College of Occupational Therapists' (1995a) guidelines on violence at work provide comprehensive information on the legal and practical aspects of violence at work and detail preventative measures that can be taken to minimize risk. Under the Health and Safety at Work Act (1974) the responsibility for ensuring the safety of employees (and students) at work rests with the employer. Policies must be in place which specify procedures for minimizing risk to staff and clients through adequate organizational arrangements, staffing levels and training.

As a student, if you are to work in an area of potential risk in hospital or in the community, you should receive clear instruction before you engage in the work, about how to minimise risk and deal with incidents if they occur. You need to be alert to circumstances which provoke threatening behaviour and take steps to avoid them. You will also need to be on your guard for your own, as well as others' safety. You will find that members of the staff team support each other if an incident occurs. Your fieldwork educator should give you instruction about your role if anything untoward should happen. In the hospital situation you should make sure that you know where 'panic buttons' are situated and the telephone number for summoning emergency help.

When working in the community where visits to clients' homes are expected you must follow the procedure for recording your whereabouts before you leave the department and for advising those concerned of your return from the visit. This ensures that someone knows where to make enquiries if you seem to be taking longer for a visit than you anticipated. Do not deviate from your plans unless you seek permission and inform appropriate personnel of your whereabouts. This is good practice as you take responsibility for your own safety. If you are on a visit in the community and feel threatened in any way, you should leave immediately. Do not even enter premises if you feel that there is danger, not just from people but also from the structural condition of the building. You should inform your fieldwork educator or other responsible person as soon as possible. If a violent incident has occurred you should take care of your own safety, seek medical advice immediately where this is necessary, and you should make a written report of the occurrence in accordance with organizational policy. You would also be advised to alert your fieldwork coordinator at the university.

LEARNING FROM OCCUPATIONAL THERAPISTS

Your fieldwork educator will almost certainly act as the primary model for your practice. You will work closely alongside him or her to begin with, observing, questioning and critiquing the interactions and interventions which occur. Eventually you will be observed by your fieldwork educator as you assume a key role with clients. Your fieldwork educator will then help you to critique your performance and identify your strengths and future needs. It is essential here that you appreciate that a critique or critical evaluation appraises strengths and limitations but does not imply criticism. A critical evaluation is intended to promote a positive and constructive learning experience.

Critiquing others' practice

Students are usually able to discriminate between good practice and that which is not so good. They are able to make choices about what features of a professional's practice to incorporate into their own work (Alsop, 1991). The concern comes when you believe that a professional is not performing as you believe he or she should, given the circumstances. You may end up criticizing (albeit in private) rather than critiquing professional performance and questioning the practice that is taking place. What should you do?

The first thing to do is to clarify your observations or perceptions. You may wish to check out the facts with the therapist concerned and ascertain his or her reasoning for actions taken. The aim is for you to try to understand what has transpired from the other person's perspective. You may find that your criticism is unjustified once you have listened to the explanation. In a professional way, you may like to put forward another viewpoint, drawing on your own understanding or experience, and to explain any difference in your perception of what happened. There are often different approaches to practice which can be readily explained, so be careful about being critical in such circumstances. Reserve your judgement. You may wish to check things out with someone else, possibly your fieldwork educator. If you feel uncomfortable about a particular approach taken, there is no reason why you should adopt it. However, you will always need to justify the approach that you do adopt, whether you are a student or an occupational therapist.

From time to time, students do come across what they judge to be poor or bad practice or even malpractice. In dealing with such situations you should maintain diplomacy and professionalism. You may need to seek guidance and support from university staff. Judgement about inadequate or inappropriate practice can be based on personal experience and become a subjective judgement, or can be based on professional knowledge and experience which has a foundation in research or well-documented, commonly held views of 'experts' in the field. Malpractice, however, contravenes the Profession's Code of Ethics and Professional Conduct (College of Occupational Therapists, 1995b). This states that under no circumstances must any occupational therapist who witnesses malpractice, whether by an occupational therapist or other professional, remain silent about it. You should speak in confidence to someone in authority as quickly as possible if you have witnessed an incident of this nature.

As students you are learning to make judgements based on sound knowledge and good reasoning. This will be expected of you. As you develop in professional life the judgements you make are likely to become more refined and be based on more sophisticated reasoning skills. You will see this explained more in Chapter 14. You may be very clear about your judgement of good and bad practice and there is nothing wrong with that. You do, however, need to be careful about seeing things in black and white, as there are always other, and sometimes better, ways of doing things. You need to remember that there are many shades of grey between black and white. Whatever you do, you need to be clear about the grounds on which you base your judgement and, where circumstances are difficult, you should seek advice from someone you trust.

Often exposure to poor practice can provide very positive learning experiences. This can seem a rather contradictory statement, but to translate the experience into learning it is important to ask why the practice is considered to be poor. Ask yourself on what knowledge or experience this practice is based, what went wrong, what were the consequences, and finally what could be done differently? Learning can result from these reflections and you should write down what you learn. This is where you might use your learning log or diary to note your observations, perceptions and reflections.

LEARNING FROM CLIENTS

Clients are an incredible learning resource, but the first thing to say about learning from clients is that in no way should clients ever be exploited for learning purposes.

They have rights, such as that of privacy, confidentiality, dignity, all of which must be preserved. Nevertheless, provided that you are honest with clients about your student status and your desire to learn from them, then listening to their experiences and insights can provide an invaluable source of information.

As you listen to clients' life stories they will become real and you will remember them vividly for a long time. The memories that you store as you discuss the stories provide a bank of material on which to draw later for reference and for helping you in your practice. The skills that you need to develop, such as interviewing, listening, checking out information, and of interpreting and integrating information are those that you would do well to develop. They are needed, not only to assist your academic studies, but also to assist you in professional practice in whatever setting you choose to work. Jenkins *et al.* (1994) note the importance of the communication process in Occupational Therapy, and Mattingly and Fleming (1994) emphasize the place of life stories in understanding the meaning of disability in clients' lives.

Learning from others

There is often concern about students having insufficient exposure to Occupational Therapy practice to be properly socialized into the profession, hence the reason for the requirement that students gain 1000 hours experience under the supervision of occupational therapists. In pursuing this requirement there can be a tendency to dismiss the learning that can take place from being exposed to the practice of other professionals. Many individuals have highly developed personal and professional skills which are used in a unique way in the process of care delivery. Individuals may be members of other professions but equally may be members of voluntary organizations, with or without formal professional qualifications. The knowledge and experience these people offer can be no less valuable, and time spent with them can provide insights into other perspectives and approaches which could be useful in professional life. If you take advantage, selectively, of opportunities to work alongside people with a different range of skills you will begin to gain a more complete picture of care from the client's perspective, and you will begin to form a clearer idea of the boundaries of Occupational Therapy and other professional groups. The skills of interviewing and listening, and of interpreting and accommodating information are just as applicable when learning from members of other professions.

PRACTISING WITHOUT DISCRIMINATION

Increasingly occupational therapists are operating in services where there is a high proportion of clients from minority ethnic backgrounds. The education of students needs to address the special needs of these clients (Colston, 1994) so that practitioners can offer services which are non-discriminatory and relevant to the different needs of clients. Efforts have been made more recently within the Occupational Therapy curriculum to address issues of difference between people from different cultures and to prepare students for work in a multi-ethnic, multi-racial society.

Representation of Occupational Therapy students, and thus practitioners, from minority ethnic groups is also increasing in the United Kingdom. Fieldwork educators have a responsibility to act as a model for students and demonstrate anti-discriminatory practice, both towards the student and towards the client. In Social Work, this requirement is much more explicit in the profession's curricular requirements and practice expectations than it is in Occupational Therapy. The Central Council for Education and Training in Social Work (CCETSW, 1995) expects qualifying social workers to practise in an ethnically sensitive way and to be able to understand and counteract the impact of discrimination. The value base relating to anti-racist, anti-discriminatory practice on which social work practice is founded becomes a model for other professions. In the practice setting there is an expectation that educators and students accept the validity of others' experiences and reality of the world as perceived by each individual, so putting the student/educator relationship on a more equal footing (Shardlow and Doel, 1992).

In the context of fieldwork education it is important that issues of race and discriminatory practice are addressed openly. It is a fairly sensitive area and frank discussion often depends on each individual's attitude towards acknowledging the level of his or her own understanding of the issues, and towards learning. This relates to both student and educator, but students are in a more vulnerable position because of the perceived 'power' relationship between themselves and the educator.

As a student, you should obviously expect to be treated fairly and with respect regardless of your colour, race, ethnic background, gender or sexual orientation, and be given opportunities equal to those afforded to any other student on placement. The employing authority will have an Equal Opportunities Policy which employees are expected to respect. Discrimination and harassment are normally dealt with seriously. Discriminatory practice and racism will also be dealt with seriously by university staff who should, as part of their own Equal Opportunities Policy, promote anti-discriminatory practice, both within the university and also in fieldwork settings.

If, as a student, you consider that you are being discriminated against, or that those involved in your education are demonstrating racist behaviour or attitudes towards you, you must take steps to deal with the matter. Some students find it easier than others to face the issue and challenge the individual concerned, others find it more daunting because of the power relationship. No student should be subjected to racism or discrimination on placement. Sometimes it does occur through ignorance or insensitivity which can usually be remedied, other times it occurs through attitude, in which case the situation is less easy to manage. You should not let the matter pass or get out of hand, because it could become intolerable and affect you personally as well as affect your studies. You should contact a tutor at your university if you feel that the situation cannot be resolved by yourself alone.

SUMMARY

The organization is the context of the learning experience. It is influenced by legislation from which the service philosophy is developed. Occupational therapists are contributors to the totality of service provision. They are often members of teams or smaller service units which are jointly responsible for the work of the wider organization. These teams or units may not be managed by occupational therapists. Learning to carry a caseload means contributing as a team member to client care. The team and clients are both resources which can be used for learning. Participating in service delivery should be undertaken within the ethical principles of the profession and within an explicit framework of anti-discriminatory practice.

REFERENCES

Alsop, A. (1991) *Five Schools Project: Clinical Practice Curriculum Development.* Unpublished report, Dorset House School of Occupational Therapy, Oxford.

Barnitt, R. (1993) What gives you sleepless nights? Ethical practice in occupational therapy. *British Journal of Occupational Therapy*, **56**(6), 207–12.

CCETSW (1995) *Assuring Quality in the Diploma in Social Work – 1.* Rules and Requirements for the DipSW. Central Council for Education and Training in Social Work, London.

Christie, B. A., Joyce, P. C. and Moeller, P. L. (1985) Fieldwork experience: Part 11 The supervisor's dilemma. *American Journal of Occupational Therapy*, **39**(10), 674–81.

College of Occupational Therapists (1995a) *Violence at Work.* College of Occupational Therapists, London.

College of Occupational Therapists (1995b) *Code of Ethics and Professional Conduct for Occupational Therapists.* College of Occupational Therapists, London.

Colston, H. (1994) Occupational therapy courses and applicants from minority groups: attitudes and feelings. *British Journal of Occupational Therapy*, **57**(10), 398–400.

Jenkins, M., Malett, J., O'Neill, C., McFadden, M. and Baird, H (1994) Insights into 'practice' communication: an interactional approach. *British Journal of Occupational Therapy*, **57**(8), 297–302.

Mattingly, C and Fleming M. H. (1994) *Clinical Reasoning. Forms of Inquiry in a Therapeutic Practice*. F.A Davis Company, Philadelphia.

Reed, K. and Sanderson, S. (1993) *Concepts of Occupational Therapy*, 3rd edn. Williams & Wilkins, Baltimore.

Robertson, L. (1995) *Problem representation*, Paper presented at the Australian Occupational Therapy Conference, Hobart, Tasmania.

Scrivens, E. (1982) Rationing – theory and practice. *Social Policy and Administration*, **16**(2), 136–48.

Shardlow, S. and Doel, M. (1992) Towards anti-racist practice teaching. *Practice*, **6**(3), 219–25.

12 Being supervised

This chapter covers:

- the supervisory relationship;
- the facilitation of learning;
- styles of supervision;
- models of supervision;
- the process of supervision.

This chapter examines in more detail the nature and process of supervision so that you can make the best use of it in practice. Most authors agree that supervision is a **process** but individual authors place emphasis on different facets of this process. As we explain below, an understanding of the nature of supervision is very important so that you can be clear about what to expect of a fieldwork educator and what part you must play in the supervisory process.

DEFINING SUPERVISION

Relationships within supervision

Frum and Opacich (1987) draw on the work of Loganbill *et al.* (1982) to define supervision as an intensely, interpersonally focused, one-to-one relationship in which one person is designated to facilitate the development of therapeutic competence in the other person. You will note that this definition focuses on the quality of the relationship between two people and the facilitative nature of the process. In contrast, Yerxa (1994) implies that the student is in a more subordinate role. She describes the supervisor as one who, by reason of his or her greater knowledge and skill, establishes a relationship which leads, teaches, supports and provides a barometer of performance for another person. This seems to imply a more directive relationship where evaluation of performance is included as part of the process. You can see, therefore, that different relationships with your fieldwork educator are possible. The quality of that relationship is sometimes dictated by the educator's experience.

A study by Christie *et al.* (1985) stated that lesser experienced supervisors expected students to take a more passive role in the relationship, whereas experienced supervisors saw fieldwork as a more collaborative venture where their role was to work

with the student. Experienced supervisors expected students to take initiative, to communicate their needs and to ensure that these needs were met. These expectations place the responsibility for learning squarely on the student although no-one would deny that the fieldwork educator has a significant role to play in the development of the student's learning. You can see that it is important to clarify both your fieldwork educator's expectations and your own expectations as to the nature of your particular relationship. You should discuss and agree this together.

Supervision as a communication process

According to the College of Occupational Therapists (1993) supervision is a communication process between supervisor and student. The process enables the student to explore and increase knowledge and understanding of professional practice and to develop and apply Occupational Therapy skills and knowledge. A number of researchers (Christie *et al.* 1985; Emery, 1984; Michael, 1976) note that the supervisory relationship thrives on good communication and interpersonal skills. A good relationship has communication as its heart because it enables a student to feel comfortable about discussing strengths, limitations and needs clearly and honestly with the fieldwork educator. Open discussion allows a fieldwork educator to gain an accurate assessment of the level of development at which the student is functioning. Good communication is valued by students (Alsop, 1991) and seen as a trait in those they call 'good' fieldwork educators (Michael, 1976). It entails a willingness to communicate, as well as demanding clarity in its process and content. Regularity of communication, especially in feedback, is required. Communication is thus an essential medium through which knowledge and skills are firstly established and subsequently developed.

Supervision as an educational process

According to Shepheard (1957) supervision is essentially an educational process which aims to help the student to use, in a professionally disciplined manner, his or her natural ability to relate to clients. In supervision, the supervisee begins to understand theoretical concepts and principles and learns how they can be used in practice. The focus of supervision here is on more than just teaching and learning. Supervision, seen as an educational process, implies much more. There is far less emphasis on the end product which Loganbill *et al.* (1982) call 'therapeutic competence', and far more on the process of learning which involves both an understanding of self and an understanding of theory and its application in practice.

Just taking stock for a moment, you can see that supervision is a multi-faceted concept which authors have described in different ways. In sum, supervision is an educational process which relies on effective relationships and open communication between student and fieldwork educator.

Facilitation of learning

Facilitating or enabling your learning is a responsibility of the fieldwork educator but inevitably this cannot be done without your cooperation. You have to participate actively in the process if any development of your therapeutic competence is to take place. In facilitating your learning the fieldwork educator will expect you to come to the supervision session well prepared and in a position to discuss recent events and experiences. Reflecting on these events and experiences will be your responsibility. You will be encouraged to think through selected experiences, reviewing them in your mind, so that you learn from what happened. The fieldwork educator may prompt you, guide the discussion and probe your knowledge and understanding, but essentially you must do the work.

As a student in the fieldwork setting you are somewhat dependent on the perceptions and capacity of your fieldwork educator to act as a facilitator of your learning. The facilitation process is successful when your fieldwork educator is able to gauge the degree of structure needed to guide your learning. There is a balance to be found between controlling your activity and allowing you some freedom to act independently in the fieldwork setting. Whatever type of relationship you find yourself in, we would still suggest that you play an active role to maximize your learning. Honest communication about your needs as well as your strengths is vital if you wish your fieldwork educator to help you achieve your aims.

STYLES OF SUPERVISION

Entwistle (1981) argues that fundamental differences in personality affect our styles of learning – our preferred way of thinking. He also suggests that approaches to teaching reflect our previous experiences with learning, therefore 'we teach as we prefer to learn'. This would suggest that fieldwork educators are likely to adopt a style of supervision which reflects their own learning style. This is fine if it is compatible with your preferred learning style, but a mismatch of learning styles between a fieldwork educator and a student could affect the quality of supervision and therefore the quality of the student's learning.

Learning style preference has been defined as the preferred mode of obtaining knowledge (Rogers and Hill, 1980). If you are not sure about how you prefer to learn then we suggest that you complete Honey and Mumford's (1992) Learning Styles Questionnaire which is to be found in their manual.

Honey and Mumford describe four learning styles: Activist, Reflector, Theorist and Pragmatist. When you have completed the questionnaire you may find yourself dominant in, or favouring one style more than others. Alternatively you may find that you demonstrate a balanced repertoire of skills across the four styles. This would indicate that you have the ability to adopt and benefit from different learning strategies according to circumstances. There is no right or wrong learning style, and everyone's result will be different. The process merely shows that different people benefit from different modes of teaching and learning.

You may be wondering how this helps us in our exploration of the supervisory process. Imagine what might happen if your fieldwork educator was quite dominant in one style of learning and you were quite dominant in another. Neither of you would be wrong, but the approaches that you choose to take towards teaching and learning may well be incompatible. Your fieldwork educator might suggest a particular strategy to facilitate your learning which might be quite unacceptable to you, or might have expectations of you in a learning situation with which you feel quite uncomfortable.

These incompatibilities often explain 'personality clashes' which arise between a student and fieldwork educator. Knowledge of learning styles, relationships and relevant teaching approaches can often minimize difficulties because adjustments can be made in the approach to teaching and learning. The ideal would be for both students and educators to recognize differences and to develop their ability to learn in different ways so that each could be flexible and use different teaching and learning strategies effectively. Different skills tend to lend themselves to different ways of learning and you may find that there is much to gain from being attentive to different methods used.

MODELS OF SUPERVISORY RELATIONSHIPS

A number of authors have written on models and styles of supervisory relationships (Ford and Jones, 1987; Gardiner, 1989; Michael 1976). Michael described three styles of supervision, two of which she categorized within an apprenticeship model and the third which centred on students' education. Although there are several models of the supervisory relationship we outline three here, the apprenticeship, growth and educational models, so that you can see the differences. It may help you to identify the nature of the supervisory relationship in which you find yourself, and so assess its potential for learning.

Apprenticeship models

Apprenticeship models emphasize what fieldwork educators have to offer from their repertoire of knowledge, skills and experience. Service commitments establish the boundaries of the experience offered in the fieldwork setting. Learning is limited to whatever transpires in the workplace as a natural consequence of service provision. The experience as an educational one is not really fostered, and only minimum regard is paid to aims, objectives and individual learning needs. Basically, you learn to do things in the same way as your fieldwork educator in that setting.

Growth models

Growth models focus on students' personal experience, growth and self-awareness in the learning situation. These models are influenced by psychodynamic psychology. There is a belief that encouraging the personal and psychological growth of practitioners is a pre-requisite to successful therapeutic practice in the future.

Educational models

Educational models operate on a different value basis. They place emphasis on students' learning, on educational aims and expectations and on course expectations.

This requires a shift in thinking and attitude for practitioners whose value system normally places clients' needs at the centre of their attention. Fieldwork educators working to this model accept the dual responsibilities of the practitioner/educator role and balance the demands of both roles, giving each the attention it requires.

Learning and personal growth will occur through all models of supervision but it is probably fair to say that the quality of learning is likely to be significantly enhanced where your educational needs are the focus of attention.

THE PROCESS OF SUPERVISION

We have explained that during fieldwork you have a designated fieldwork educator who supervises both your placement and your practice. Overall, the process of supervising your placement means that your fieldwork educator will take responsibility for:

- promoting an environment in which you can learn;
- managing your fieldwork experience;
- facilitating your learning;
- providing you with necessary support and constructive feedback on your performance;
- evaluating your performance with regard to competence.

We have already stressed the educational nature of the process. The focus is on your experience and your learning so you should view supervision as a positive educational experience which is essential to your professional growth. In fact many therapists continue to ask for, and have, supervision sessions throughout their early years of practice. More experienced therapists may continue to have supervision, perhaps with someone who is not necessarily a member of the same profession but who nevertheless can still facilitate their professional growth.

We have also suggested that you have a role to play in making the most of learning through fieldwork. In earlier chapters we highlighted the responsibilities you must take to make the fieldwork experience a success. In summary:

- you should prepare well for the placement;
- act professionally at all times;
- play an active role in all dimensions of service provision and administration;
- adopt an enquiring approach to learning;
- take initiative and responsibility for performance, both in learning and in client care.

Taking an active, rather than passive role will give you plenty to talk about in supervision sessions.

Exploring practice under supervision

The fieldwork experience gives you a chance to explore practice through observation, participation, by asking questions and through reflecting on your work. This is why the relationship you have with your fieldwork educator is important and should support open communication. Some fieldwork educators are more aware of your need to ask questions than others. There are those educators who perceive questioning to be a threat and avoid presenting you with an opportunity to clarify your thoughts. Others are uncomfortable about, or just not used to, describing their practice to others (Mattingly and Fleming, 1994). They tend to hold back, perhaps not seeing the value to you of relating aloud what they are doing, and why. As an exercise, it is quite beneficial if an educator describes what he or she would do, or would have done, with **your** client. Talking about different ways of working with the same client has more advantages than selecting another client for comparison. When you start to contrast practice, however, choosing and discussing a second person often helps.

Some educators behave with students in the same way as their educators behaved with them during their training, which may mean that they act as **teacher** and **tell** you about practice instead of acting as the **facilitator** of your learning. There is a subtle difference in the communication patterns between a student and teacher and between a student and facilitator. A teacher adopts a more hierarchical relationship with the student and tells the student about practice. Acting as a facilitator, an educator **interacts** on a similar plane as the student and at the student's level of professional development. The facilitator explains practice in words and methods that are understandable to the student.

The facilitatory relationship encourages two-way enquiry and dialogue about practice. Apart from the knowledge you gain as a student, the therapist can often learn from you, for example about the latest theories or models of practice that are being taught at university. Learning therefore occurs for both of you.

There are things you can do to make sure your questions are addressed satisfactorily during fieldwork. At the beginning of the placement ask your fieldwork educator when you will have a chance to ask questions. Should you:

- ask at the time the question arises?
- keep a notebook and write down questions and ask later?
- try to find out answers from other sources?
- ask for a short informal question session once a day?
- try to fit in question time when it can be managed such as travelling between appointments or at lunch?

Learning comes from enquiry. It is therefore important to establish when this enquiry might happen so that your learning needs can be satisfied. Often this is overlooked. Fieldwork educators have been known to say of their student that he or she 'has bothered me all day long with questions, it is getting on my nerves!' Agreeing a time for questions ensures that your needs are met at a time convenient to you both.

Evaluating practice

A whole chapter is devoted to assessment so we shall not explore the concept here in very much detail. We do, however, want you to see how the assessment of your practice is dealt with in the process of supervision through self-monitoring and formal feedback on your performance.

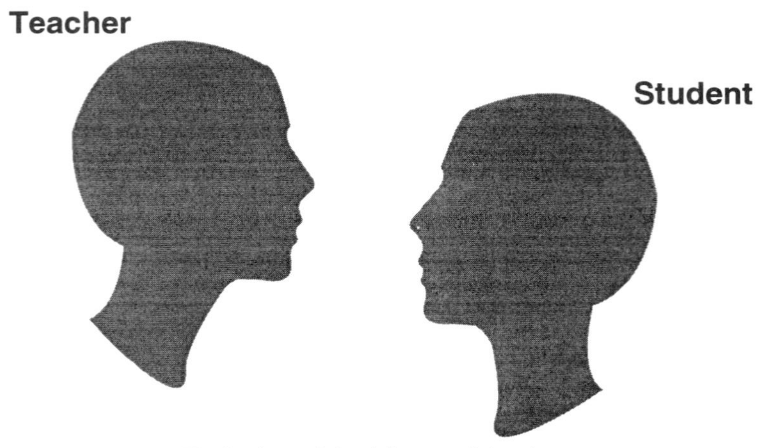

- Relationship hierarchical
- Facts are told
- Questions respond to telling
- Communication is more one way
- Encourages passivity
- One party learns

Figure 12.1 A teacher telling

The guide to your education will be your learning contract, and the guide to your overall performance in practice will be the university assessment (evaluation) form. Together these documents indicate the expectations of you during fieldwork. You should consult both of them regularly. The university requirements, which include the requirements of the professional body, are non-negotiable. The learning contract, however, is negotiable, and should be updated at regular intervals throughout the placement to reflect learning and progress towards meeting the university's expectations. Before we go on to examine informal and formal supervision, we consider how you might monitor your own performance and receive feedback as part of the learning process.

Self-monitoring

The ability to monitor and critique your own performance is essential to you as a practitioner. You need to develop self-evaluation skills necessary for examining your own practice against established standards as part of quality monitoring and audit. Making critical judgements about the effectiveness of your personal perfor-

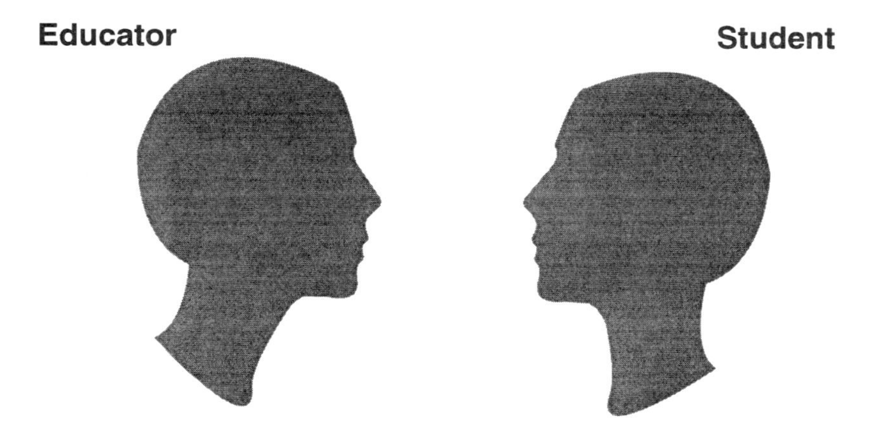

- Relationship on similar plane
- Discussion at student's level of professional development
- Encourages two way enquiry
- Both parties learn

Figure 12.2 An educator facilitating

mance through reflection and open discussion will help you to develop these necessary skills. Some placements have an evaluation form with a Likert-type scale, usually graded 1–5, where you are asked to judge your own performance as a means of self-monitoring in relation to personal skill development and placement goals.

Your need for feedback

Feedback is different from both evaluation and criticism. Henry (1985) defines the term feedback as a form of non-judgemental communication which can be both formal and informal. The different elements of this interaction are shown in Figure 12.3.

Some educators can be reluctant to give feedback for fear that students will lose confidence, so you may need to ask for it. Feedback should take into consideration your thoughts as well as your feelings and your reflections on the situation. Feedback, if given properly, stimulates learning. It is only from finding out what others think of your ideas and performance that you can form a picture of how you are operating, and you can set their opinions against your own. Try to listen carefully to what is being said when feedback is given to you. Avoid denying the issues raised or jumping in too quickly with a 'yes ... but ...' response. You will learn more from 'hearing' what your fieldwork educator has to say.

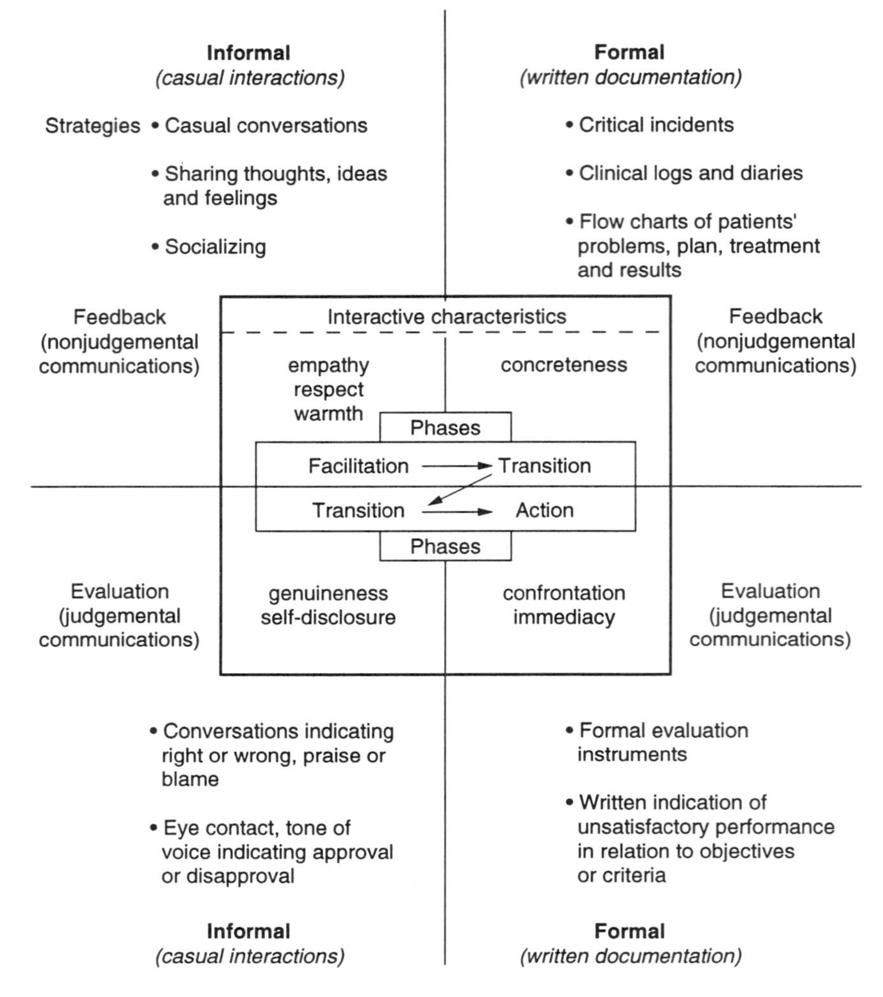

Figure 12.3 Formal and informal feedback and evaluation
Reprinted with the permission of the American Physical Therapy Association

Source: from Henry, J. (1985) Using feedback and evaluation effectively in clinical supervision: model for interaction characteristics and strategies, *Physical Therapy,* **65**(3), 354–57.

Feedback should not be confused with praise:

Oh you are doing really well on this placement!

This sort of remark is non-specific and contributes to a false notion that **everything** you are doing is good. Feedback should be very specific and should be directed at something tangible that you have done. For example:

> ... I liked the way you responded to Mrs ... when she became so upset this morning. The way you touched her arm seemed to really comfort her.

This form of feedback pinpoints an incident, reinforces what you did, and describes the result of your action. If your fieldwork educator is not giving you feedback which relates to specific incidents then ask for more details or specific examples from your practice. The fieldwork educator must be able to justify the comments he or she makes about your performance or behaviour and this is usually done by reference to incidents which have happened. These are referred to as 'critical incidents'. Don't forget that feedback is also a two-way process. You might have a need to give feedback to your fieldwork educator, formally or informally as the system allows.

Informal supervision

Informal discussions about service activity and client care can take place at any time during your fieldwork experience, sometimes several times a day. They are part of the general process of integrating your educational needs with service delivery and ensuring that you understand practice. Some of these discussions may take place before, during and/or after a session with a client. Sometimes the client is invited to participate in discussions which are enacted for your benefit. These methods are intended to assist your learning and allow you to gain first-hand insights about the client's circumstances so that you can begin to understand the nature of this particular Occupational Therapy intervention.

Still informally, but away from client contact, your fieldwork educator may encourage more reflective dialogue about a client's situation and the therapeutic process in order to promote your active participation in reasoning, decision-making and learning. After you have interviewed, or interacted with, a client your educator may give you immediate feedback on your performance, but may also highlight issues which need further consideration in a more formal supervision session.

Informal supervision tends to take place in an *ad hoc* way between sessions, during refreshment breaks or while travelling between appointments. It is usually governed by service commitments but nevertheless it is time well spent and it allows for immediate feedback and discussion.

Formal supervision

Formal supervision, by contrast, should occur regularly at pre-arranged times in a quiet environment free from the distractions of service delivery. Supervision sessions can last between one and two hours and form an essential feature of the placement and supervisory process. These sessions are a pre-requisite of your fieldwork education and should be treated with respect by both you and your fieldwork educator.

Formal supervision should be used for four main purposes:

1. reflection, feedback on, and dialogue about practice;
2. review of the achievement of learning goals;
3. revision of the learning contract, until the next supervision session;
4. exploration of practice issues to a deeper level of understanding.

We have already addressed three of the elements of supervision noting how reflection and dialogue facilitates your learning and stressing the importance of updating the learning contract frequently to reflect current learning needs. Now we would like to take time to examine how the supervisory process can help you to gain a deeper understanding of different facets of professional practice.

Formal supervision is a time for problem setting and for appraising options for problem resolution, sometimes in a hypothetical way but often drawing on real case stories as a foundation for debate and clinical reasoning. Formal supervision is a time for exploring practice, a time for learning, where the real objective is your professional growth.

For these supervision sessions to be successful your fieldwork educator needs to be able to assess and work at the developmental level at which you are operating. We will explain a little about developmental stages so that you can become aware that there is a developmental process to your education and so that you can understand the implications that it has for your practice.

Stages of development

Gardiner (1989) proposed that students operate at three levels of development.

1. Where they focus on the content of learning, believing there to be a right and wrong way of doing things.
2. Where they focus on process, recognizing the diversity in practice and playing an active part in constructing meaning from their experience.
3. Where they demonstrate versatility in learning, adopting learning strategies appropriate to the circumstances.

Your development depends on you being able to shift your thinking and learning to a level where you are able to move between content and process learning as appropriate to the situation.

If both you and your fieldwork educator recognize and approach supervision in accordance with the known level of your performance, learning will be maximized because expectation of performance and actual performance will be at the same level. If expectation and actual performance are at different levels then difficulties normally arise. A mismatch in communication can occur, leading to confusion and possibly to conflict. Provided that your fieldwork educator is aware of these stages of development, he or she can use that knowledge in his or her approach to supervision.

Similarly Schwartz (1984) describes a three stage model of clinical supervision which reflects a student's developmental stage. This draws on Loevinger's (1977) work on stages of development and focuses on problem-solving and the student's use of rules to guide practice. At an early stage of development students tend to be limited in their capacity to generate solutions to problems, but as they begin to operate at a higher level of understanding they show a greater capacity to deal with complex issues and to see a greater number of alternatives for problem-solving. Students will first conform to rules, then challenge rules which do not fit with their value system until they can understand them better. Students functioning at the highest level are able to accept multiple viewpoints and they have an ability to understand the complexities of problematic situations.

Problem setting, clinical reasoning, creative thinking and problem-solving are needed for successful therapeutic practice so it is reasonable to expect you to develop these abilities as part of your education. Dealing with complex problems is a skill which is developed over time. Some students manage it sooner than others, some only manage it in certain fields of practice, but not others. Although problem-solving relies on a knowledge base it is essentially a process and depends on the development of sophisticated processing skills in reflection and reasoning and is highly dependent on the context and your actual understanding of the organization and of the needs of clients with whom you are working. This is why we spend time in this book explaining how you can develop these skills through active engagement in learning and practice.

Successes and failures

The formal supervision session is the time for exploring your successes in practice and for gaining some deeper understanding of how they occurred. But it is also a time for exploring mistakes and failures in practice. A critical analysis and evaluation of problems and events can often turn negative experiences into positive learning. In analysing practice it is a good idea to ask yourself:

- what happened?
- what went well, or what was good about the experience?
- what did not go so well, or was not so good?
- what would you want to do differently?
- what would others want you to do differently?
- what have you learnt from the experience? (Coles, 1991)

These questions are the essence of experiential learning and can be used to think through any problems or experience in personal or professional life.

Deeper understanding of professional practice can be developed in supervision by your fieldwork educator:

- testing, probing and verifying your knowledge;
- challenging your assumptions;
- enabling you to search for and identify other solutions for problems;
- prompting you to think through the consequences of your plan or action;
- enabling you to relate principles and theoretical concepts to actual practice;
- helping you to transfer your knowledge of one situation and apply it to another.

The supervision session

We conclude by looking at the actual process of a formal supervision session in which we encourage you to take a very active role. Table 12.1 summarizes the responsibilities that you can take in the process and shows how you might prepare for, participate in and learn from the supervision session.

Table 12.1 The process of a supervision session

Prior to the supervision session you should:

- review your learning contract
- review the work you have undertaken to date
- identify and note your achievements
- note what you have learnt from your different experiences
- review the university's assessment form; carry out a self-assessment of your performance
- identify further learning needs
- note any concerns you have, and topics for discussion in supervision
- make an agenda
- undertake any preparatory reading

During the supervision session you should:

- agree the agenda with your educator
- take initiative and participate equally in the discussion
- take the lead in reviewing your performance to date, expressing both strengths and limitations
- explore any issues that have given you special cause for concern
- give feedback to your educator on strengths and limitations of supervision, noting any consequence for you as a student
- specify particular needs which you have identified, and prioritize them
- establish which needs might be met, and how
- ensure that your learning contract is updated
- agree a course of action for the next few days
- clarify your responsibilities in the course of action

After the supervision session you should:

- review the session
- make notes of the event and of your learning from the session
- undertake supplementary reading to clarify issues and consolidate learning
- prepare to fulfil the action plan

You will note particularly that you need to spend time on preparatory activities. This is part of the process of you maintaining control of learning which we discussed earlier. It is also a reason for ensuring that supervision sessions are planned in advance. There may be times when your fieldwork educator will attempt to 'fit in' supervision on the spur of the moment. However useful the session, it will not allow you to prepare, you are less likely to feel in control and the session may seem rushed. By all means take advantage of the time for discussion but try to book another time soon afterwards with your fieldwork educator so that educational issues can be addressed more thoroughly and when you are properly prepared. We have stressed all along that the supervisory process is essentially an educational one. It is up to you and your fieldwork educator to ensure that your educational aims are fulfilled.

SUMMARY

Recent definitions of supervision suggest that it is an educational process which depends for success on a good relationship being developed between fieldwork educator and student and where open communication can facilitate learning. An appreciation of the effect of similarities and differences in learning style, and an awareness of different models of supervision can assist understanding of the supervisory process. Feedback, both informal and formal, from a fieldwork educator is an essential feature of supervision but the student is also expected to take responsibility for participating actively in the supervisory process and for monitoring his or her own performance in practice.

REFERENCES

Alsop, A. (1991) *Five Schools Project: Clinical practice curriculum development.* Unpublished report, Dorset House School of Occupational Therapy, Oxford.

Christie, B. A., Joyce, P. C. and Moeller, P. (1985) Fieldwork experience, Part II: the supervisor's dilemma. *American Journal of Occupational Therapy*, **39**(10), 675–81.

Coles, C. (1991) *Protocol for Reflecting on Practice.* Presentation at a conference, 16.10.91, Dorset House School Of Occupational Therapy, Oxford.

College of Occupational Therapists (1993) *Guidelines for Assuring the Quality of the Fieldwork Education of Occupational Therapy Students.* Standards, Policies and Proceedings Statement on Fieldwork Education SPP165. College of Occupational Therapists, London.

Emery, M. J. (1984) Effectiveness of the Clinical Instructor. *Physical Therapy*, **64**(7), 1079–83.

Entwistle, N. (1981) *Styles of Learning and Teaching.* John Wiley & Son, Chichester.

Ford, K. and Jones, A. (1987) *Student Supervision.* Macmillan, Basingstoke.

Frum, D. and Opacich, K. (1987) *Supervision: the Development of Therapeutic Competence*, The American Occupational Therapy Association, Rockville, MD.

Gardiner, D. (1989) *The Anatomy of Supervision.* Society for Research into Higher Education/Open University Press, England.

Henry, J. N. (1985) Using feedback and evaluation effectively in clinical supervision. *Physical Therapy*, **65**(3), 354–7.

Honey, P. and Mumford, A. (1992) *The Manual of Learning Styles,* 3rd edn. Peter Honey, Ardingly House, Linden Ave., Maidenhead, Berkshire. England.

Loevinger, J. (1977) *Ego Development: Conceptions and Theories.* Jossey-Bass. San Francisco. CA. In Schwartz, K.B (1984) An approach to supervision of students on fieldwork. *American Journal of Occupational Therapy*, **38**(6), 393–7.

Loganbill, C., Hardy, E. and Delworth, U. (1982) Supervision: a conceptual model. *Counseling Psychologist*, **10**(1), 3–42.

Mattingly, C. and Fleming, M. H. (1994) *Clinical Reasoning: Forms of Inquiry in a Therapeutic Practice.* F.A Davies Company, Philadelphia.

Michael, G. (1976) *Content and Method in Fieldwork Teaching.* Unpublished PhD thesis, University of Edinburgh, UK.

Rogers, J. C. and Hill, D. J. (1980) Learning style preference of bachelors and masters students in occupational therapy. *American Journal of Occupational Therapy*, **34**(9), 789–93.

Schwartz, K. B. (1984) An approach to supervision of students on fieldwork. *American Journal of Occupational Therapy*, **38**(6), 393–7.

Shepheard, E. (1957) Function and practice of supervision in psychiatric social work. *British Journal of Psychiatric Social Work*, **4**(2). In Michael, Content and method in fieldwork teaching. Unpublished PhD thesis, University of Edinburgh, UK.

Yerxa, E. (1994) Techniques of Supervision. In *Guide to Fieldwork Education*, American Occupational Therapy Association, Inc., Bethesda, MD.

13 Practising as a professional

This chapter covers:

- the concept of professionalism;
- professional judgement, including ethical and legal reasoning;
- professional socialization and professional development.

Have you given any thought to what **professionalism** is all about? As you embark on fieldwork education this is a good time to reflect on the concept of professionalism and what it might mean for you. During your fieldwork education you will be expected to conduct yourself professionally, gain professional experience, draw on professional knowledge, develop professional expertise, exercise professional judgement and be assessed on professional competence. These factors may be said to be the constituents of professional performance and practice. Your socialization into the profession can depend on your ability to develop professionalism, that is, to absorb and use the various dimensions of professional knowledge and attitudes in professional practice.

As Foster (1992) points out, professionalism goes beyond the possession of a knowledge base and cognitive skills, it includes the way in which an individual conducts him or herself. It embraces professional demeanour, clinical competence, personal behaviour and professional development. It reflects values in daily practice, responsibilities for maintaining competence and professional standards, and obligations to respect clients' rights and wishes. Let us examine the term **professional** a little more.

PROFESSIONS AND PROFESSIONALS

Bond and Bond (1994) define a profession as an occupation with the following attributes:

- the use of skills based on theoretical knowledge;
- education and training in these skills;
- the competence of professionals ensured by examinations;
- a code of conduct to ensure professional integrity;

- performance of a service that is for the public good;
- a professional association that organizes members (p. 262).

Foster (1992) also suggests that a unique body of knowledge is pertinent to the practices and beliefs of a profession and that a sound theory base should underpin its philosophies and values. Commitment is needed by the membership to adhere to the profession's practices and beliefs and to further its development, and that continuing education maintains standards in the light of change.

The Code of Ethics and Professional Conduct for Occupational Therapists (College of Occupational Therapists, 1995) makes explicit professional expectations and the type of behaviour of which the profession disapproves. According to Mosey (1983) a code of ethics guides the actions of practitioners and serves as a contract with the society that the profession serves. As a member of the profession, the practitioner pledges to abide by the Code of Ethics and Professional Conduct and use it to guide his or her behaviour with clients and colleagues. A summary of the expectations of a professional is given in Table 13.1. Many of the points made are drawn from the work of Baly (1984).

Table 13.1 Expectations of a professional

A professional is an independent practitioner who:

- is working largely unsupervised
- is governed by the requirements of a professional body
- uses competence and skill more than the ordinary person
- provides a unique service to clients
- works to a 'contract' between society and the profession
- has a responsibility to change as the needs of society change
- does not abuse the privileges which society affords (client abuse; withdrawal of labour)
- puts the client first
- maintains confidentiality
- works within the law
- respects the rights of individuals
- upholds anti-discriminatory principles in practice
- takes responsibility for own performance
- knows personal limitations
- maintains oneself as competent in practice
- evaluates one's own practice and performance
- collaborates with others in providing a service to clients

Source: Baly, M. E. (1984) The hallmarks of a profession. In *Professional Responsibility*, 2nd edn. John Wiley & Sons.

Gaining membership of a profession makes certain demands of people in terms of education, training and examination in the principles and processes of that profession's practice. Commitment to the profession's philosophies and beliefs is a requirement of membership, as is the expectation that members continue to develop their skills and maintain their competence to practise. Competent performance involves making professional decisions and judgements in practice backed up by sound clinical reasoning.

During fieldwork, under guidance of qualified staff, you will be put into situations where you will have to make judgements – simple ones at first, and eventually more complex ones. The fieldwork experience provides opportunities for you to develop the reasoning skills necessary for making professional judgements.

PROFESSIONAL JUDGEMENT

Professional judgement is not easy to define. Discussions around the topic (Dowie and Elstein, 1988) refer to decision-making in the light of uncertainties, probabilities, ethics, legalities, economics, scientific analysis and intuition but no specific definition is given. Eraut (1994) attempts a definition by referring to professional judgement as 'the wise decision made in the light of limited evidence by an experienced professional'. Abercrombie (1989) however, suggests that judgement is not the **result** of action but the **process** of observing and thinking and, we would argue, reflecting, which involves:

- reacting to information;
- ignoring some of it;
- seizing some of it;
- interpreting it in the light of past experience in order to make as good a guess as possible about what is going to happen, giving due consideration to the consequences;
- reflecting on the knowledge available.*

(*added by the authors)

One succinct definition of professional judgement which has been coined by an Occupational Therapy student is based on a range of definitions. Memie Shillingford (personal communication, July 1995) suggests that professional judgement is:

> the ability to make rational decisions based on acquired knowledge, experience and expertise which demonstrates competence and integrity, instilling confidence and trust in clients and which is justifiable under scrutiny.

According to Dowie and Elstein (1988) there are two questions to be answered:

1. how **do** clinicians make judgements?
2. how **well** do clinicians make judgements?

The first has already been addressed. In summary, this is to do with collection and interpretation of data and, as Schon (1988) points out, it is to do with setting the problem before trying to solve it. Problem-setting means converting a problematic situation into a problem by making sense out of the situation. If problem-setting is inaccurate, the problems addressed may be the wrong problems!

The second question about the quality and acceptability of judgements is addressed below. The debate is continued in Chapter 16 which explores how therapists progress from being **novices** to being **experts**.

Good judgements, it seems, depend on good data collection, good data processing and defining the problem accurately. This mirrors what occupational therapists do as they establish the nature of the client's problem, clarify needs and expectations, goals and priorities with the client, and decide which problems to work on first. The quality of professional performance is assured by ensuring that those who address clients' needs are knowledgeable and skilled in the required range of techniques (Ovretveit, 1992). Ovretveit suggests that it takes a professional to judge whether the best treatment was given in any situation even though the client may be involved with decision-making. It therefore places the responsibility for good judgement squarely on the professional who becomes the facilitator in the collaborative therapeutic process.

Making good professional judgements requires an individual to draw on a range of clinical, ethical and legal reasoning skills and can involve some economic analysis. The quality and acceptability of judgements however may be a matter of debate since ethical principles help determine the way in which judgements are reached.

Ethics in professional practice

Ethics is the branch of philosophy that examines voluntary human action to determine what types of activity or actions are right and wrong (Kyler-Hutchinson, 1988). Bioethics is the application of general ethical theories, principles and rules to problems of therapeutic practice, healthcare delivery and medical and biological research (Beauchamp and Childress, 1983). Key ethical principles are said to be those of autonomy, veracity, non-maleficence, beneficence, confidentiality and justice (Francour, 1983, cited in Barnitt, 1993). The beliefs that individuals hold about what is right and wrong underpin ethical theories and principles.

Table 13.2 Ethical considerations

	PRINCIPLE	
Beneficence	*Respect for human dignity*	*Justice*
Freedom from harm Freedom from exploitation Benefits from research The risk/benefit ratio	The right to self-determination The right to full disclosure Issues relating to the principles of respect	The right to find treatment The right to privacy

Occupational Therapy is underpinned by a value-base which believes in choice for, and empowerment of, clients to enable them to make informed decisions about their future. Kyler-Hutchinson (1988) suggests that an understanding of bioethics is important for occupational therapists because it makes them aware of their patients' need for autonomy and self-determination in making decisions. Collaboration between practitioners and clients in practice is thus needed to facilitate informed decision-making by the client. To begin with, however, operating collaboratively with clients may not be easy for students who often need time to develop the skills and confidence to practise in this way. The use of role play and practice with peers or your fieldwork educator can assist in the development of your confidence. At least some of the important scenarios can be dealt with in this way.

At first you are likely to use your fieldwork educator as a model and to learn from observing other practitioners as they seek to empower clients. Reflecting on your observations and evaluating the process of client-centred practice can help your learning. You then need to try things out for yourself in the relative safety of the fieldwork placement. Working collaboratively with clients often means making judgements about how to select information and present it appropriately to them and how to enable clients to make decisions for themselves. As you will see in the next chapter, sound clinical reasoning skills will assist the process.

Legal reasoning

All professional practice is undertaken within the boundaries of the law. Sometimes specific Acts of Parliament guide therapists' work, such as the Chronically Sick and Disabled Persons Act 1970 and subsequent Disabled Persons (Services Consultation and Representation) Act 1986. Laws relevant to all employees such as the Health and Safety at Work Act 1974 and the Data Protection Act 1984 also apply. At all times, however, both criminal and civil law guide the judgements that are made with, or on behalf of clients. Since no occupational therapist is above the law, legal, as well as ethical reasoning has to inform professional judgements. Although working within the law does not guarantee good judgements, poor judgement may constitute negligence, which is addressed below.

UNPROFESSIONAL BEHAVIOUR AND MISCONDUCT

Very rarely on fieldwork does a situation arise when a student is considered to be unprofessional. Codes of professional conduct are explicit in their expectations and students as well as qualified staff are expected to respect them. Minor matters, or 'one-off' occurrences involving a student's unprofessional behaviour are normally dealt with promptly by the fieldwork educator. The student is counselled and the matter quickly resolved.

In more serious cases of a student's misconduct or when unprofessional behaviour is a consistent problem, matters are dealt with in accordance with university regulations. Fieldwork educators have a right to suspend a student from the fieldwork setting, although only university staff can normally suspend a student from a programme of study. Fieldwork educators will ensure that their clients or colleagues are not put at risk by the student's presence, conduct or behaviour. Often course regulations permit the fieldwork educator to warn students verbally or in writing about unprofessional behaviour or minor breaches of codes of conduct as part of the disciplinary procedure. Any student who has been informed that he or she has breached a code of conduct should obtain a copy of the regulations and procedures for dealing with such matters from the university and would be well advised to get in touch with their union. Major breaches of such codes are serious and can lead to a student being required to leave the course.

NEGLIGENCE

Students are no different from any other person in that they owe 'a duty of care' to the people with whom they work. This may be clients, carers or colleagues, or indeed anyone. Any harm that is caused to another person as a result of failure to exercise that duty of care could amount to negligence. Dowie and Elstein (1988) state that one test is to ask the question 'was this action reasonable to this particular person at this particular time?' (p. 36).

As students, you are at your most vulnerable when on fieldwork placement and need to be very sure about what you can and cannot do. The law on negligence covers both 'acts' and 'omissions' of an individual which result in harm to another person. This means that if you **do something** or if you **fail to do something** which causes harm to someone (anybody and not just a client) that act or omission could be construed as negligent. It would be for the court to decide, if matters got that far.

Although the incidence of negligence is fairly low it needs to be discussed. At the same time it should be noted that in everyday practice where judgements are involved there is always an element of uncertainty and always an element of risk. Provided that practitioners and students go about their business in good faith and with reasonable regard for safety, problems are unlikely to occur.

This is where we must reinforce that you should know and act within the limits of your competence, check with your fieldwork educator regarding tasks about which you feel uncertain before taking the responsibility, report to your educator any situation where you consider a person to be at risk, and record all your dealings with clients.

If a dangerous or untoward incident occurs you should act professionally at all times and deal with the matter at hand. It is impossible to state explicitly what you should do in any situation, this will involve your own judgement, but as a general guide the following advice may be helpful. Unless your own life is at risk you should attend to anyone who is injured or in danger and call for assistance straightaway. You should make no claims as to the cause of the incident and keep your opinions to yourself. The incident will have to be reported in accordance with the organization's policies and procedures and, if serious, may need to be investigated further. If you are being investigated then you should seek legal advice before you say anything to anyone.

Immediately after the event you should write down what happened. You should note the day, date, time and place of the incident, who was present, and what you saw anyone do or heard anyone say. You should confine yourself to facts that you know to be true and avoid opinions, inferences and assumptions. You should make the record as detailed as you can. You should sign and date it and keep it safe for future reference. You should not leave it with your fieldwork educator or anyone in the placement, but keep it yourself. Sometimes actions for negligence are brought before the court many years after the event and you will need your notes to refer to. You should take the same action for any incident you witness even if you were not a major player in the event. Above all you need to protect yourself in such situations. These comments are not intended to alarm you as incidents are quite rare. The advice is intended to serve as a clear guide just in case you should find yourself in such circumstances.

ETHICAL DILEMMAS IN FIELDWORK

Barnitt (1993) notes that students return from placements with a variety of concerns which can be described as ethical or moral dilemmas. Sometimes these are matters which might be considered within a legal context. Other issues, such as the 'fairness' in the distribution of limited resources and risk-taking often present as problems, not only for students, but for qualified practitioners as well. Sometimes ethical dilemmas result from problems which require decisions to be made according to different, often conflicting, ethical principles. Two of the main ethical theories are Utilitarianism and Deontology. Utilitarian theory takes account of the consequences of actions and seeks to maximize benefits and minimize harm. Deontology focuses on respect for the rights and wishes of an individual without consideration of the consequences of action (Barnitt, 1993).

Often, doctors and administrators draw on different ethical theories in their work especially when allocating resources to client care. This can create tensions in times of financial constraint (Cassidy, 1988). Unpalatable decisions about the use of scarce resources have to be made (Brody, 1983) and occupational therapists can be caught up in the dilemma. Rationing, including prioritizing, has to occur (Scrivens, 1982). Some clients will have a proportion of their needs met, others none at all. Dowie and Elstein (1988) acknowledge the dilemma but note that health care professionals often dismiss the relevance of economic analysis in their work which can lead to poor clinical judgements. Sound judgements, it seems, cannot be made without thinking about resource issues, both for the individual client and the client population as a whole. This is why many services are making explicit the priority cases with which they will deal. The Code of Ethics and Professional Conduct for Occupational Therapists gives guidelines on accepting referrals and initiating treatment where resources may not allow basic standards to be met (College of Occupational Therapists, 1995).

These are not the only ethical dilemmas presented to students. There are many, and few have easy answers. Some relate to confidentiality or loyalty, others to malpractice. Most are likely to cause concern. Knowing whether to raise a matter for discussion can be a problem for students and sometimes it is not clear to whom the matter should be addressed. As we have said before, it can help to talk about dilemmas. If you find yourself in that position you will need to judge whether to approach your fieldwork educator, someone else in the same service or a member of the university staff. Our advice is to talk about it with someone, perhaps your mentor, rather than harbour it and hope it will go away.

PRACTISING AS A PROFESSIONAL

So far, this chapter has addressed the issue of professionalism and the more formal matters of acceptable and unacceptable professional behaviour. But there are many more facets to professional performance. Students have to 'become' professional and to be **socialized** into the profession, which is an ongoing process not one which ceases on qualification. This means that as you progress through your education you will need to take on board the values, attitudes and demeanour required of an occupational therapist. It is not just about you developing a knowledge base and relevant skills but about you taking on the complete professional role, and all the responsibilities which go with it. Your professional education, and in particular your fieldwork education, will play a significant part in your professional socialization.

Professional socialization

Becoming a professional means accepting the value base of your chosen profession and using personal qualities in a way which is consistent with the profession's philosophies and beliefs. To become an occupational therapist you will need to develop sound interpersonal skills and a sensitivity towards the needs of others. In particular, you will need to adopt the profession's unique approach and learn to use yourself as a medium in the therapeutic process. The Occupational Therapy profession draws heavily on the use of occupation and activity as a basis for its practice, but the personal qualities of the occupational therapist are essential to the process of improving a client's situation.

Those who are to develop into expert occupational therapists are likely to have the personal qualities and attitudes needed for the role before they enter the profession. Professional education, of which fieldwork education is a major part, will help students to develop their personal strengths and use them effectively in client care.

As an Occupational Therapy student, you will be required to become well-versed in the professions's **core** practice – its core skills, processes and activities. That means knowing what is unique about the profession's approach, and the techniques and processes used by its members. Some qualifying occupational therapists find this a problem as they see so much overlap between Occupational Therapy and other professions. Others are quite clear about the unique dimension that occupational therapists bring to a client's care.

People often talk about **core skills** in Occupational Therapy practice but this is not always a helpful phrase in distinguishing the Occupational Therapy profession from others. Health and social care workers from other professions often claim to use the same core skills in their practice. The difference in use is often difficult to articulate and demonstrate. Occupational therapists do, however, use a **core approach** in their work. This is a unique way of thinking about a client's situation which incorporates the different components of self-care, productivity and leisure and acknowledges the client's 'world' as he or she sees it. The **meaning** which clients give to the different elements of their life then guides the formulation of an action plan which occupational therapists and clients work on together.

In fieldwork situations you will need to be alert to the way in which occupational therapists in different settings use this approach. In being exposed to, and evaluating occupational therapists' approach and performance in practice, you will be noting which values underpin their work, which skills they draw on, and how they use them to bring about positive change in a client's situation. This will play a significant part in your professional socialization. You will absorb these characteristics and integrate them in your own work as part of the learning process.

Working in settings where no occupational therapists practise

In the last paragraph we argued that exposure to occupational therapists and their work is essential for professional socialization. This cannot be denied. However, the profession is in a constant state of change and is in a unique position to be able to cross boundaries and develop its practice in environments where occupational therapists are not yet employed. Had there never been situations like this, occupational therapists would never have moved away from 'occupying' (in a therapeutic sense of course!) people in hospital undergoing long-term treatment and care. Pioneers advanced the profession's practice into other situations. The delivery of services in a variety of community settings is the mode of the moment. Many of these services are run neither by health nor local authorities but by private enterprises and charitable trusts. They are often very effective in meeting the specific needs of selected clients, and have much to offer as learning environments for students.

Some would argue that placing a student in an environment where there is no occupational therapist will not help the student to socialize properly into the profession. It will leave the student confused and uncertain about Occupational Therapy practice. This is one point of view which is important to acknowledge. A student who is uncertain about Occupational Therapy practice may not be helped in their professional development by being placed in such an environment. However, we pride ourselves in our profession on the fact that we see and treat people as unique beings and acknowledge each individual's strengths and limitations. Not all Occupational Therapy students are the same. Some may be very capable of moving into new surroundings, integrating with other professionals and showing what occupational therapists can do. These will be the students who are clear in their mind about the profession's 'core approach' and are personally able to cope with more ambiguity. Students who are unable to contemplate working in non-traditional environments will be right to insist on placements where occupational therapists are close at hand.

As you progress through your course you will learn a good deal about yourself and your capabilities. Your fieldwork placements will help shape your thoughts and may help you to determine your future career movements. Often, although not exclusively, the last placement in a programme of study is one where a little more freedom is exercised and you may be allowed to choose the environment in which to practise your skills before finally qualifying. There is scope to venture into new settings. This is the time to compare other approaches with the way in which occupational therapists approach the work. This is the time to be alert to new ideas which can be absorbed quite comfortably into the occupational therapist's domain. This is the time to be proactive, to learn from others but also to demonstrate what occupational therapists can do in such situations. Socialization into the profession of Occupational Therapy will still take place, but in a different way.

PRACTISING WITHOUT DISCRIMINATION

As occupational therapists we espouse the belief that everyone is an individual with a unique set of circumstances, problems and needs. One of the most difficult aspects of practising as a professional is being able to suspend one's own standards and perceptions about the way in which people should live, in order to work effectively with clients and meet the needs they have in a way which is acceptable to them.

Increasingly we are working in a multi-ethnic, multi-cultural society and it is imperative that we learn to operate without discrimination, without giving offence to the people we meet and without making judgements about people's lifestyle. This means engaging actively in learning about different cultures and seeking relevant information especially from people whose lifestyle is significantly different from our own. Local ethnic community groups may be contacted for advice. One way of building up knowledge of working with different client groups and with people with different conditions, problems and needs is to create a portfolio of professional experience (Alsop, 1995).

THE PROFESSIONAL PORTFOLIO

Brown (1992) defines a portfolio as

> a collection of evidence which demonstrates the continuing acquisition of skills, knowledge, attitudes, understanding and achievement. It is both retrospective and prospective as well as reflecting the current stage of development and activity of the individual (p. 1).

The word is developed from the Latin *portare* and *folium* interpreted as meaning to carry leaves. Artists use them to show work which they have previously completed to potential employers. The idea is that a collection of material is brought together in some orderly format to provide evidence of learning and ability.

A portfolio is one way of recording and evaluating your experiences and of documenting your learning which has taken place during your professional career, for future reference. You might do this to show evidence of learning and professional updating, or in order to present the material for accreditation of prior learning (APL) as part of an academic award (Alsop, 1995). On the other hand you might just create a portfolio for personal use. One way of recording information is in a learning log which we explained in Chapter 10.

Developing a portfolio which captures professional knowledge and experience is not only a practical thing to do during fieldwork to serve as a reference for the future, it is a professional way of documenting learning, of bringing together evidence of professional development and of showing how you have used your learning in practice. Sometime in the future this may be a requirement of continued State Registration to practise as an occupational therapist. Forming the habit of keeping a portfolio while you are a student will provide you with a basis on which you can build during the rest of your professional career.

SUMMARY

There are many expectations of people who claim to be professional and who have a desire to practise professionally to meet the needs of their clients. Professional performance and practice requires commitment to the profession's philosophy and beliefs, and the ability to practise legally, ethically, safely, non-discriminately and with sound judgement. There is a responsibility placed on the individual to ensure that he or she develops and maintains competence to practise within the profession. This process is initiated in the educational programme, where fieldwork plays a significant part. Ongoing learning is then required and needs to be demonstrated. Professional experiences and evidence of ongoing learning can be documented in a professional portfolio for future reference and as a record of personal achievements.

REFERENCES

Abercrombie, M. L. J. (1989) *The Anatomy of Judgement*. Free Association Press, London.

Alsop, A. E. (1995) The professional portfolio: purpose, process and practice, part 1: Portfolios and professional practice. *British Journal of Occupational Therapy*, **58**(7), 299–302.

Baly, M. E. (1984) *Professional Responsibility*, 2nd edn. John Wiley & Sons, Chichester.

Barnitt, R. (1993) What gives you sleepless nights? Ethical practice in occupational therapy. *British Journal of Occupational Therapy*, **56** (6), 207–12.

Beauchamp, T. L. and Childress, J. F. (1983) *Principles of Biomedical Ethics*, 2nd edn. Oxford University Press, New York. In K. Hutchinson, Ethical reasoning and informed consent in occupational therapy. *American Journal of Occupational Therapy*, **42**(5), 283–7.

Bond, J. and Bond, S. (1994) *Sociology and Health Care*, 2nd edn. Churchill Livingstone, Edinburgh.

Brody, B. (1983) *Ethics and its Application*. Harcourt Brace Jovanovich, New York. In R. Hansen, Ethics is the issue. *American Journal of Occupational Therapy*, **42**(5), 279–81.

Brown, R. A. (1992) *Portfolio Development and Profiling for Nurses*. Central Health Studies Quay Publications, Lancaster.

Cassidy, J. (1988) Access to health care: a clinician's opinion about an ethical issue. *American Journal of Occupational Therapy*, **42**(5), 295–9.

College of Occupational Therapists (1995) *Code of Ethics and Professional Conduct for Occupational Therapists*. College of Occupational Therapists, London.

Dowie, J. and Elstein, A. (eds) (1988) *Professional Judgement, A Reader in Clinical Decision Making*. Cambridge University Press, Cambridge.

Eraut, M. (1994) *Developing Professional Knowledge and Competence*. The Falmer Press, London.

Foster, M (1992) *A Basis for Practice*. In A. Turner, M. Foster, S. Johnson (eds), *Occupational Therapy and Physical Dysfunction*, 3rd edn. Churchill Livingstone, Edinburgh.

Francour, R. (1983) *Biomedical Ethics*. John Wiley, New York. In R. Barnitt, What gives you sleepless nights? Ethical practice in occupational therapy. *British Journal of Occupational Therapy*, **56**(6), 207–12.

Kyler-Hutchinson, P. (1988) Ethical reasoning and informed consent in occupational therapy. *American Journal of Occupational Therapy*, **42**(5), 283–7.

Mosey, A. C. (1983) *Occupational Therapy: Configuration of a Profession*. Raven Press, New York.

Ovretveit, J. (1992) *Health Service Quality: An Introduction to Quality Methods for Health Services*. Blackwell Scientific Publications, Oxford.

Schon, D. (1988) From technical rationality to reflection in action. In J. Dowie and A. Elstein (eds), *Professional Judgement: A Reader in Clinical Decision Making*. Cambridge University Press, Cambridge.

Scrivens, E. (1982) Rationing – theory and practice. *Social Policy and Administration*, **16**(2), 136–48.

Developing reasoning skills

14

This chapter covers:

- clinical reasoning processes; inductive and deductive reasoning;
- frameworks and perspectives of practice;
- narrative framing and case stories;
- clinical reasoning and Occupational Therapy: the therapist with the three-track mind.

Clinical reasoning is about thinking and talking about the way you work and giving the reasons for what you do. Clinical reasoning forms the basis of all therapeutic practice and underpins problem-solving, so it is crucial to understand what it entails. Once you have mastered clinical reasoning ideas you can start to develop the processes that will help you become proficient at reasoning, and this will improve your practice.

INTERNALIZING EXPERIENCE

As therapists mature in experience their ways of reasoning develop but often in an *ad hoc* manner. Studies have found that while experience is necessary to become an expert, not all therapists with experience have developed expert reasoning powers (Ryan, 1990). Knowledge and reasoning is usually internalized by therapists rather than being voiced aloud. Experienced therapists are not used to talking through what they are doing, their thinking remains private. Mattingly and Fleming (1994) call this implicit or tacit knowledge and they believe that it needs to be made public so that others can learn from it.

CLINICAL REASONING

The classical interpretation of reasoning is that it is the process of applying scientific logical thought which determines, and then accounts for, initial ideas, hypotheses or problems. Effective reasoning will therefore depend on the foundation of knowledge which forms the base from which solutions are drawn.

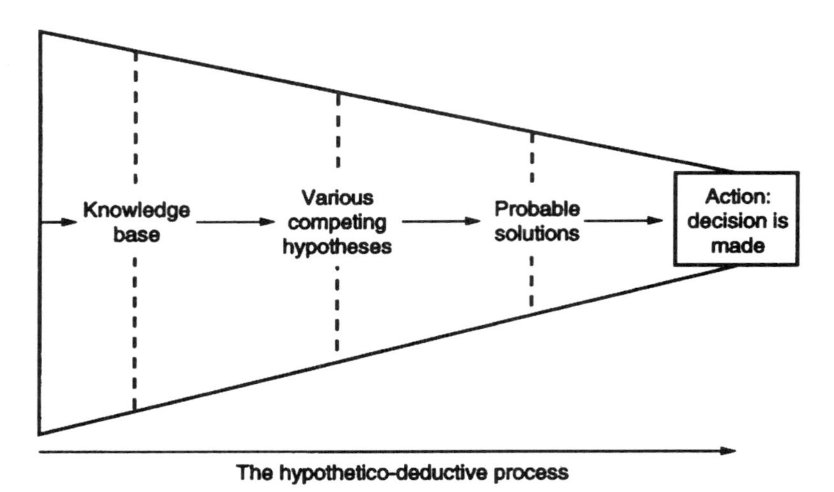

Figure 14.1 Competing hypotheses

However, it is now being accepted that clinical or professional thinking may be a more fitting construct to describe the process that we are talking about, because thinking through and about professional problems requires more than that implied in the definition above.

INDUCTIVE REASONING

You will read in the literature about terms such as brainstorming, creative thinking, inductive reasoning, parallel processing, and lateral thinking. These terms all describe the process of developing breadth of ideas from which possible solutions to problems may be found. This is a process called induction or inductive reasoning. Mattingly (1989) and Ryan (1990) both found that experienced therapists in the course of their work automatically considered a range of options before they decided what to do. Therapists without much experience did not seem able to do this. Students tend to take a narrower approach, problem-solving only from existing information. Thinking widely and inductively is an important skill to develop as you need to find ways of generating ideas and possible solutions to problems. You should write down all the options you can think of for addressing a particular problem and then discuss the merits and limitations of each idea. Figure 14.2 shows this inductive pattern of thought.

You can see from Figures 14.1 and 14.2 that the potential for generating options is greater if you think inductively.

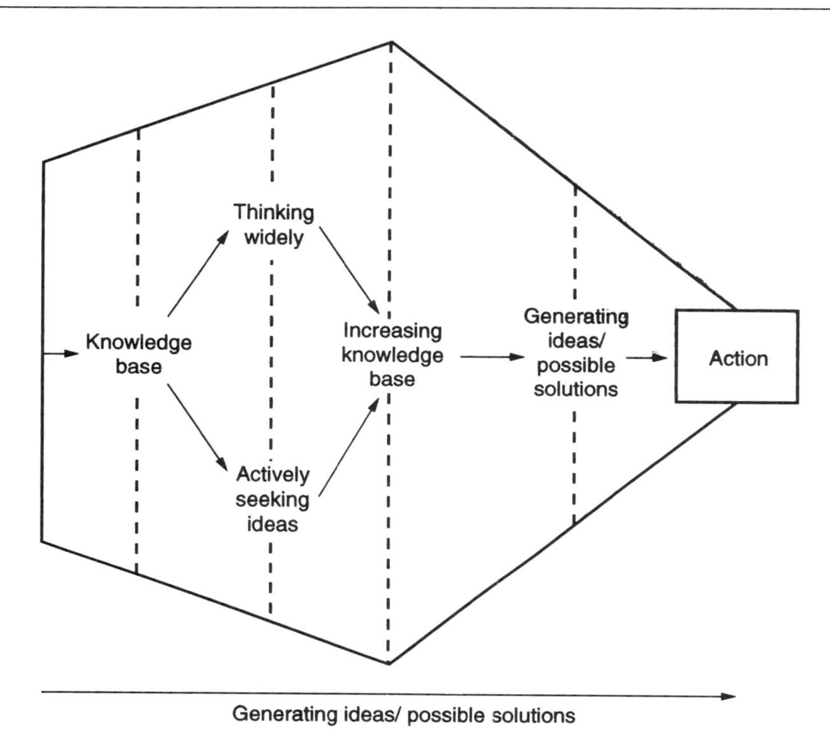

Figure 14.2 Inductive thought

DEDUCTIVE REASONING

It is only when inductive reasoning is complete that you should start to narrow down your thinking into problem solving, to do what the literature calls hypothetico-deductive reasoning (Higgs, 1990). You examine the different hypotheses or options, systematically working through the information in order to determine some agreed course of action. All reasoning should be accompanied by critical thinking and collaborative reflection to maximize the probability of a successful outcome to problems addressed. The next chapter deals with different ways of reflecting to enhance your learning and reasoning skills further.

In this chapter we are making the following assumptions.

1. professional problems are complex and involve many issues;
2. clinical reasoning is not simple and does not follow a straightforward, linear procedural path;
3. clinical reasoning cannot be taught as a separate subject as it is embedded in practice. It can be facilitated by creative means.

According to Higgs and Jones (1995) reasoning develops in an ever increasing upward and outward cyclical spiral as the understanding of clinical problems grows.

You might note from Figure 14.3 that with additional insights, problems are reformulated many times before they are solved.

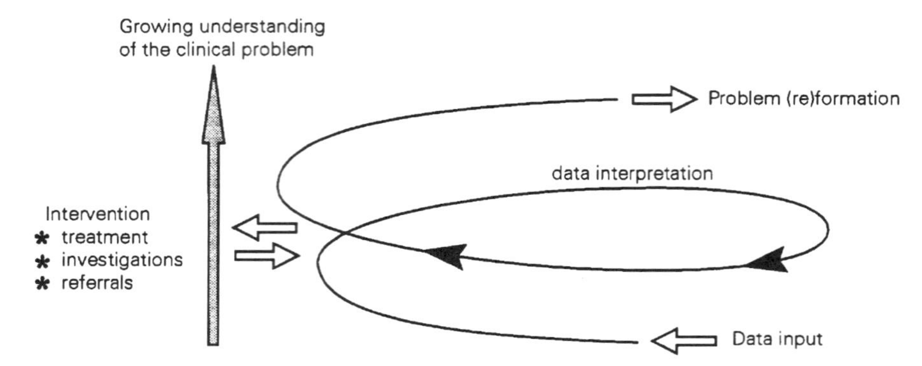

Figure 14.3 Clinical reasoning within a loop
Reprinted with permission
Source: Higgs, J. and Jones, M. (eds) (1995) *Clinical Reasoning in the Health Prfessions.* Butterworth-Heinemann Ltd, Oxford

PUTTING YOUR FRAMEWORKS TOGETHER

You need to be aware of the different frameworks or structures that influence the setting in which you are working. You should also be aware that putting a frame around any kind of thinking can actually inhibit, limit and possibly simplify too much the information that needs to be considered in practice. It is because of these potential constraints that we have titled this section frameworks. Trying out different frameworks can help order a therapist's thinking, although the frameworks will vary according to the area of practice in which the therapist is working. No framework is uni-dimensional and each has the power to increase in breadth and depth as other factors become known.

Growth comes with experience, with further knowledge and with a deeper understanding of the significance of other perspectives. In this sense, clinical reasoning is inextricably bound to the context of the practice setting. By examining a succession of frameworks, as if taking layers off an onion, you can build up your foundation of knowledge.

BUILDING YOUR OWN FOUNDATION OF KNOWLEDGE

Let us look at three frameworks which consider different perspectives of practice. Each is presented in a different way. Some may appeal to you more than others, and there is always overlap. The first looks at the wider context of practice, the second examines the knowledge base on which you build your practice and the third gives one example of a way of working with a client. Your foundation of experience thus moves from the wider scene to the actual focus of therapeutic work. Most people, because they are anxious, make the mistake of working with a client before they have considered wider issues. This can limit vision and reasoning and thus inhibit problem-solving ability.

You might use the following exercises to help you to develop your reasoning powers. You can carry them out alone, with your peers or with your educators. You might even try to bring everyone's ideas together and synthesize them for your own use.

WIDER CONTEXTS OF PRACTICE

Figure 14.4 illustrates some of the wider contexts that you need to think about for each placement. The diagram is a useful way of considering them together. Start with the outer layer and work your way down to the centre, first discussing, and then writing down, as much information as possible.

FRAMING THE KNOWLEDGE YOU NEED TO KNOW

The second framework is one where you examine the professional or propositional knowledge base needed for the area of practice in which you are working. This exercise demands more detail than you might think. For instance, if you are working on an orthopaedic ward you might identify 'splinting' as the knowledge you require, but you must also specify whether the splints are dynamic or static, what types of splints are made and what kinds of materials are used.

The framework shown in Table 14.1 was developed by an American Occupational Therapy Association (AOTA) Task Force in 1993 and it was specifically designed for a neonatal unit. This example tends to focus on medical procedures because of the nature of the unit, but you could adapt the headings to suit your area of practice. Use the headings that are applicable and insert others as necessary. Discuss the knowledge base with different people until you are satisfied with the information you have collected. Sections could include:

1. specific definitions used in the setting;
2. client information;
3. family and social structure;
4. work environment;
5. professional and personal characteristics.

Table 14.1 expands on knowledge which might usefully be specified.

You will see that the exercise requires considerable depth of thought but by doing it before and during your placement you will discover a greater richness and diversity of knowledge.

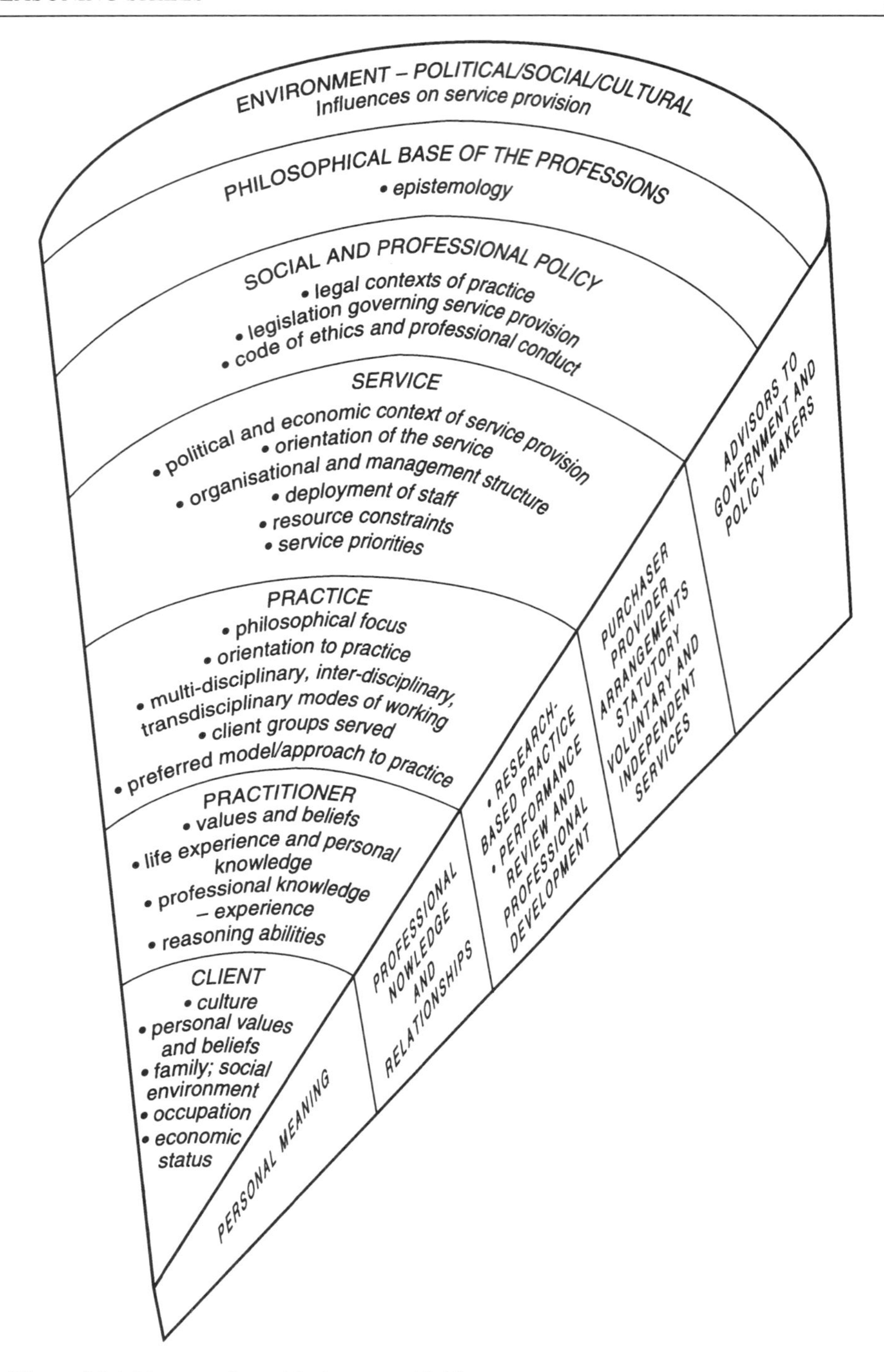

Figure 14.4 Frameworks: widening your thinking

Table 14.1 Examining your knowledge base

Specific definitions used in the setting	Client information	Family and social structure	Work environment	Professional and personal characteristics
List	• **Medical knowledge base** terminology procedural principles precautions complications pathophysiology risks precautions prognosis • **Specific knowledge base** procedures and skills effects controls • **Influencing factors** preceding onset during post condition • **Knowledge of unique factors** the development of the course the abilities and vulnerabilities of the clients the inter-relationships between medical and development factors • **Knowledge of approaches and theories** when to use them • **Specific skills** practical interactional professional (formulating interventions) • **Inter/multi professional plans and discharge**	• **Family systems** • **Learning styles suitable for family education programmes** • **Client/family interactions** • **Transitions from practice setting to home** • **Specific skills related to the family** cultural values attitudes interests strengths priorities preferred communication styles skills they need to develop • **Interactions and interpretations** • **Adaptation in the intervention processes**	• **Physical environment** equipment procedures input of procedures (timing, intensity, duration) • **Social environment** • **Non-contingent input from other persons working in the setting** • **Knowledge of organizational culture** philosophy of care roles and responsibilities and functional positions of personnel the influence of stresses communication patterns spoken and unspoken rules of behaviour effects of environment performance • **Specific skills in adapting environment** assessment of environment intervention strategies/education influencing philosophy of care assessment of intervention and revision of plan	• **Synthesizing research findings and new information** • **Ability to observe** • **Ability to bring about change** • **Understanding inter-personal skills** • **Academic interest and commitment** • **Provisions of education programmes** • **Insight into professional limitations** • **Ability to value and collaborate with other team members** • **Ability to articulate one's values, attitudes and reasonings**

Source: adapted from The American Occupational Therapy Association Task Force (1993) Knowledge and skills for occupational therapy practice in the neonatal intensive care unit. *American Journal of Occupational Therapy,* **47**(12), 1100–5

INTERPRETING PRACTICE

Studies have highlighted the difficulties that students experience in analysing, synthesizing, interpreting and evaluating the knowledge gained at university. Higgs and Jones (1995) believe that knowledge alone is not enough, it must be combined with cognition and metacognition. Cognition is about understanding the knowledge which you have acquired and metacognition is the ability to monitor your thinking processes in order to:

> detect links and inconsistencies between the clinical data and existing clinical patterns or expectations based on prior learning, to reflect on the soundness (accuracy, reliability, validity) of observations and conclusions and to critique the reasoning process itself (for logic, scope, efficiency, creativity, etc.) (p. 7).

Higgs and Jones believe there must be a harmonious interaction between all these elements.

To help you gain an understanding of these factors, and how they link together and apply to your work, you could set up a focal group. You could discuss a client who has completed his or her programme and been discharged. Members of the group could talk about their own contribution to the client's programme saying what each thought, said and did. As a group you could then examine the experience using the two frameworks above. Through critical questioning, you could put all the factors into some kind of perspective. Even then you are each likely to interpret the information in a different way. Alternative strategies are always possible.

NARRATIVE FRAMING IN THE WORKING RELATIONSHIP

The last framework which we would like you to consider will enrich your understanding of the dynamics of the therapeutic relationship between yourself and your client. It is called narrative framing and it was first proposed by Mattingly (1991) Her background was in anthropology which explains some of the different perspectives and terminology used in this work. Narratives have subsequently been used in other studies to deepen therapists' understanding of life from their clients' perspective (Kautzmann, 1993; Peloquin, 1993). There are different ways of looking at this framework. You could, for instance, visualize the narrative as an arch over the client's life. Figure 14.5 shows that you need to consider where the client sits in relation to a projected lifeline.

If your therapeutic sessions are with a child then they will fall towards the early part of the line, whereas for an older person they will be further along. If you think of that person as the central character in a book you can begin to form a story or narrative about that person's life. Some educators (Esdaile, personal communication, 1992) use this narrative method with students from the beginning of undergraduate studies. Students report that they humanize their interventions because of it.

Try this exercise yourself. Look at where your client is positioned in his/her life, as if opening a book. Try to imagine from the information that you have, what has

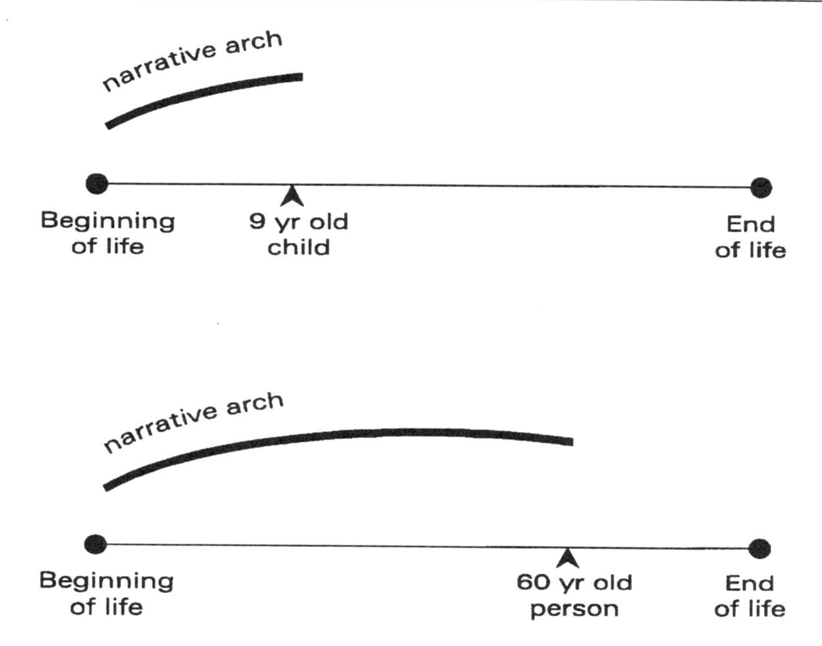

Figure 14.5 Narrative lifelines

gone on before. This should help you to identify questions to ask of the client and the kind of information to seek out. This exercise might also highlight what is significant for that person so when you choose activities to work on, they will be personally meaningful for the client. This will then lead you to examine what you are doing in the therapeutic session. Therapeutic sessions should mirror those aspects of that person's life on which you have agreed to work. You will see that the narrative continues in sessions as you try, through a mix and match of intervention strategies and skills, to work on meaningful activities that are part of that person's lifestyle. The narrative develops as circumstances change or new knowledge becomes available. Working in this way should enable you to increase an individual's participation in therapy.

Look carefully at Figure 14.6. It shows how you can personalize practice, and how time, or temporality, affects what you choose to do. Having completed the previous exercise, you should understand and be able to monitor your knowledge base. Look at the strategies and the skills that you have chosen to work on and follow your plans through systematically.

Therapists often say that a client is 'not motivated' to work in therapy. This is often because the client's and therapist's narratives are not the same and the person is not really interested in what is on offer. You need to be acutely aware of how your client is reacting to the session and use intervention strategies that will move things forward, wherever possible. In order to do this you must also have

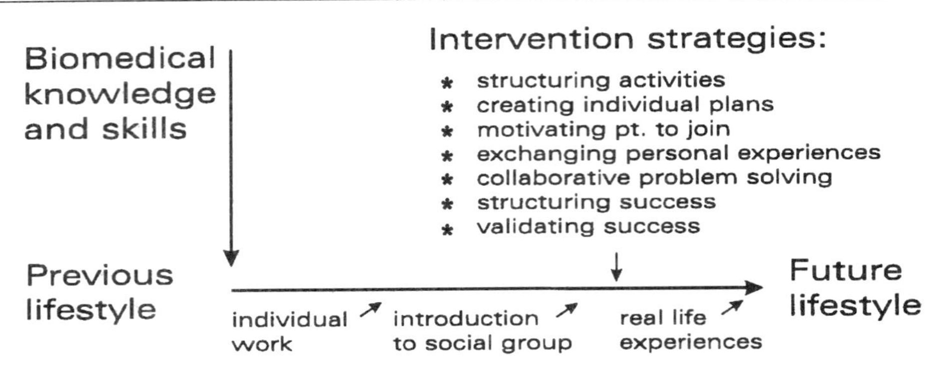

Figure 14.6 The temporal process of occupational therapy treatment: narrative framing

some appreciation of the future chapters in that person's life story. The ability to make a collaborative story and to see some picture of the client in the future, is a skill that needs to be developed. Even experienced therapists find this difficult (Ryan 1990). It is worth noting that this form of narrative is entirely different from thinking about the prognosis of the disease or disability, it entails much more. Thinking narratively ahead in this way may even prompt a review of a therapeutic programme, especially one planned for a client with major long-term problems. The picture of the future will depend on the expectations of both you and the client.

Using the language of narrative framing, the information about a client is called a **case story** rather than a case study which tends to have a more medical focus, and is much more dry. If you want to gain more understanding of the difference we suggest you read the work of Oliver Sacks. In a recently published book, Sacks (1995) quotes Father Brown who writes:

> when the scientist talks about a type, he never means himself, but always his neighbour ... so far from being knowledge , it's actually suppression of what we know ... I don't try to get outside the man I try to get inside (p. xv).

We hope that these three frameworks give you ideas for innovative ways of working and consequently, for thinking and reasoning. For those who would like to know about other frameworks and ways of using them, we recommend the work of Rogers and Holm (1989 and 1991) which is about functional assessment and diagnostic reasoning. The next section explains Mattingly and Fleming's study and shows ways of putting all this information together.

CLINICAL REASONING IN OCCUPATIONAL THERAPY

The definitive study in clinical reasoning by Mattingly and Fleming explored how occupational therapists in a physical rehabilitation centre in Boston, USA, actually worked. Cheryl Mattingly was the principal investigator and she used ethnography and action research methods to study the therapists. Ethnography is a research method used extensively by anthropologists who study other cultures; in this case it was the occupational therapists. Mattingly watched occupational therapists as they engaged in work, listened to their explanations, shared their formal and informal discussions and videotaped their practice. The action research involved the therapists in the study so that they became participants in the research. Viewing the videotapes of their work the occupational therapists explained their reasons for doing and saying the things they did. They then shared these findings with another group of therapists who challenged their thinking and suggested other perspectives and ideas that might have been tried. In this way, individual therapists became aware of a multitude of other ways of working and their sensitivity towards the client's experience increased.

Fleming, an Occupational Therapy educator, joined the project and proposed the idea that these therapists were thinking and working in three different ways, in parallel **tracks**. She called this 'the therapist with the three track mind' (Fleming, 1991). We describe each track first and then show you how they all fit together.

The top track is called the **procedural** track. This track focuses on the disability or on knowledge of the conditions that are being addressed and an image is formed in the mind. For example, if you were treating a person suffering from multiple sclerosis you would recall what you had learnt about that condition. You would know about the actual physiology, about the severity and prognosis of the disease, the length of time the person had had it, and the course of the problem. You would consider the different problems that you might expect, the ways you might identify them and what you might find out. Figure 14.7 shows the images in this track in detail.

You can see that this way of thinking is closely aligned to the 'Occupational Therapy process'. It is not totally linear because you consider a range of problems, assessments, findings and evaluations, and not just one.

The bottom track is the **interactional** track. This name can be misleading as it is about much more than interaction. This track is about forming an image in your mind, but this time the image is of the person. You **humanize** the condition that you thought about in the procedural track. Let us continue with our example of the client with multiple sclerosis.

Even before you meet the client you will probably have some idea of what to expect because of what has been derived from the procedural track. You might decide to look at medical notes to find out the person's sex, age, where they live, and how long the person has had the problem. You would form another image in your mind and you would probably start to link it with the first. Even if you decided not to look at the notes you might still hear something from staff, relatives, or from others who live or work with the client. Slowly an image will form about how that client is managing in his/her environment. As you meet and exchange information with others who know the client, this image will become stronger. Figure 14.9 highlights the main features and images which are formed in this track.

Finally, a decision has to be made about what to do. This may involve making small decisions about what to do next in the session but these decisions will be set within a larger image of how the clients might progress in the next few weeks or months. This track is called the **conditional** track as there is uncertainty in your

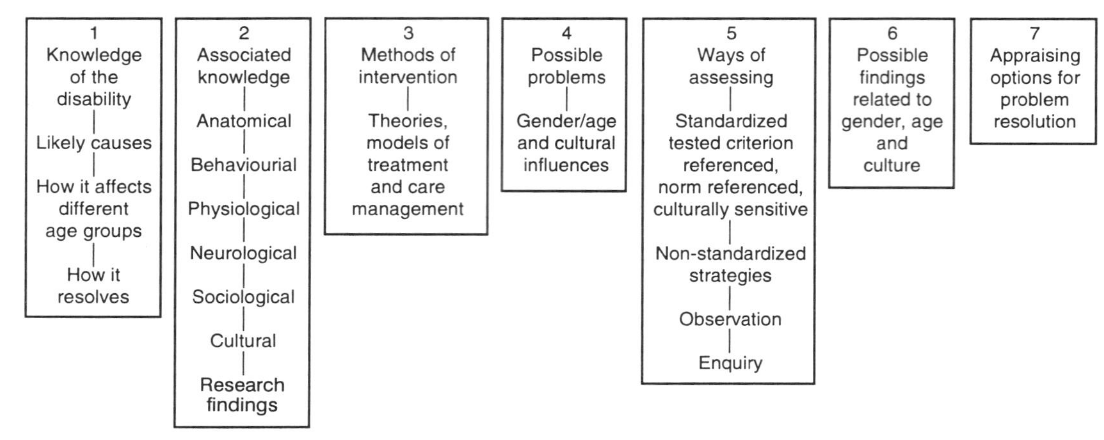

Figure 14.7 Procedural reasoning

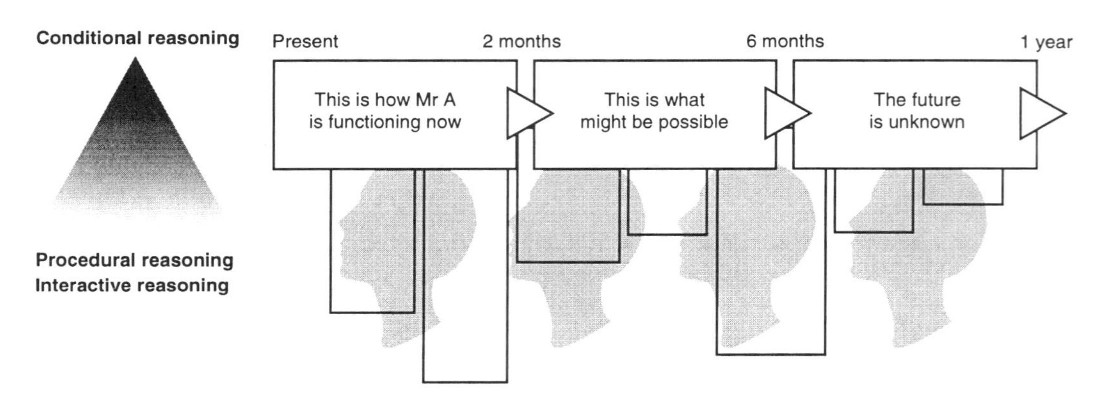

Figure 14.8 Conditional reasoning

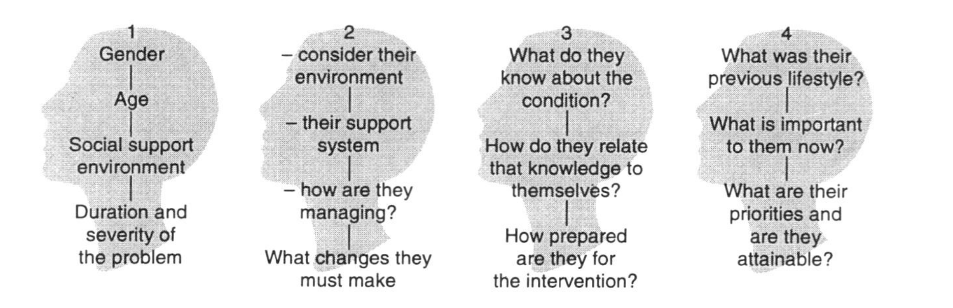

Figure 14.9 Interactive reasoning

mind about the results that may occur. Nevertheless this conditional image shown in Figure 14.8 will guide you.

This track is a synthesis of the knowledge accessed from the other two tracks and, as you can see from the composite diagram of **three track reasoning.** It is a dynamic process.

Now let us look at Fleming's (1991) description of the three-track mind shown in Figure 14.10. You will see that, not only is the process dynamic, but your thoughts go back and forth constantly between the three tracks. You can see arrows going backwards and forwards between the top and bottom track which feed into, and out of, the middle track. Therapy sessions will change according to what happens within them. The art or craft of becoming an expert therapist depend on how creatively and judiciously you can use these tracks and defend your decisions.

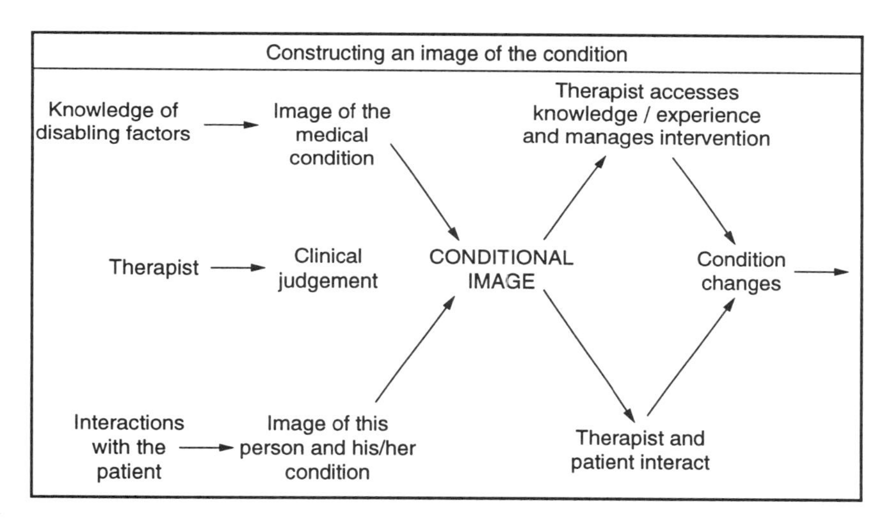

Figure 14.10 The three-track mind
Reprinted with permission from Maureen Hayes Fleming, 1991.

PUTTING IT ALL TOGETHER

Try to think of an example of someone you have worked with, or have watched with another therapist. Try to apply the thinking along these three tracks. You might want to apply it line by line and then put it all together, either by yourself or with the help of your fieldwork educator. At the beginning of this chapter we suggested that most experienced therapists tend to internalize their own knowledge. We have found that many experienced therapists work in the interactive track straight away because they have synthesized the information from the procedural track and tucked it away in their memory. As a student, you will need to bring information from the procedural track to a conscious level in order to help you think in this way. Many therapists have great difficulty doing this but practising with your fieldwork educator can help. According to Boud (personal communication, 1994) knowledge can be likened to a suitcase. You know it all, but you have to unpack it, item by item, in order to understand how it is packed together.

WAYS OF DEVELOPING YOUR REASONING

Earlier in this chapter we gave you guidelines so that you could start to create your own foundation of experience and so begin to think and reason. Working through these frameworks should help strengthen your cognition which is all about understanding, interpreting and monitoring your knowledge. We then suggested some ways of putting this cognition into practice. Finally we suggest ways of developing your skills.

If you followed the last exercise with the three track mind you will have considered one client. You will have experienced and noted the things that went well and identified the things that could have been done differently. You are stacking up these experiences for yourself like books on a shelf. Cohn (1988) refers to this as your mental library of stories. Having considered and worked through your thinking and reasoning with one client you should now do the same with another person with a similar condition, but perhaps someone from another age group or someone who behaves and copes in a different way. Working through this reasoning process helps you to become aware of differences and to consider, through discussion, how you can adapt your way of working to take account of them. You should discuss these processes with your fieldwork educator, with other professionals and with any peers who may be on placement with you. Most importantly, wherever possible, you should talk about this process with your client.

This is how you start to work 'artistically' and how you learn to individualize your interventions and tailor them to the needs of each client. Remember the advice of Sacks about humanizing therapy. Boston (1995) writes of him, 'Sacks is always learning from his patients, marvelling at them, widening his own understanding and ours.' The study of clinical reasoning tells us not only about how we work at present, but also about how we might use other perspectives in our work with clients and become truly responsive to each individual's real needs.

SUMMARY

This chapter has explained the terms and processes of clinical reasoning and noted its importance as the basis of professional practice. Examples and frameworks are given to enable students and therapists to work together to explore the knowledge base needed for practice and ways of analysing and synthesizing information to inform practice. The chapter notes how frameworks used in different environments might limit, but can also enhance, understanding of the client's situation. It advocates the use of case stories as a means of increasing awareness of the client's experience and his or her participation in therapy. The three track clinical reasoning process is explained as a means of integrating knowledge and what is known about the client at a personal level to inform decision making and the planning of an individualized therapeutic programme.

REFERENCES

AOTA Neonatal Intensive Care Task Force (1993) Knowledge and skills for occupational therapy practice in the neonatal intensive care unit. *American Journal of Occupational Therapy*, **47**(12), 1100–5.

Boston, R. (1995) cited on the back cover of O. Sacks, *An Anthropologist on Mars*. Picador: London.

Cohn, E. S. (1988) Fieldwork education: shaping a foundation for clinical reasoning. *American Journal of Occupational Therapy*, **43**(4), 240–4.

Fleming, M. H. (1991) The therapist with the three track mind. *American Journal of Occupational Therapy*, **45**(11), 1007–14.

Higgs, J. (1990) Fostering the acquisition of clinical reasoning skills. *New Zealand Journal of Physiotherapy*, December, pp. 13–17.

Higgs, J. and Jones, M. (eds) (1995) *Clinical Reasoning in the Health Professions*. Butterworth-Heinemann, Oxford.

Kautzmann, L. (1993) Linking patient and family stories to caregivers' use of clinical reasoning, *American Journal of Occupational Therapy*, **47**(2), 169–73.

Mattingly, C. (1989) *Doing with patients: occupational therapy as a collaborative practice*. Paper presented at a mini-conference on clinical reasoning, Baltimore, MD.

Mattingly, C. (1991) The narrative nature of clinical reasoning. *American Journal of Occupational Therapy*, **45**(11), 998–1005.

ÿ™Mattingly, C. and Fleming, M. H. (1994) *Clinical Reasoning: Forms of Inquiry in a Therapeutic Practice*. F.A. Davis Company, Philadelphia.

Peloquin, S. (1993) The depersonalisation of patients: a profile gleaned from narratives. *American Journal of Occupational Therapy*, **47**(9), 830–7.

Rogers, J. and Holm, M. (1989) The therapist's thinking behind functional assessment. In C. Royeens (ed.), *Assessing Function*. AOTA Self Study series, American Occupational Therapy Association, Rockville, MD.

Rogers, J. and Holm, M. (1991) Occupational therapy diagnostic reasoning: a component of clinical reasoning. *American Journal of Occupational Therapy*, **45**(11), 1045–53.

Ryan, S. E. (1990) *Clinical Reasoning: A Descriptive Study Comparing Experienced and Novice Occupational Therapists*. Unpublished master's thesis; Columbia University, USA.

Sacks, O. (1995) *An Anthropologist on Mars*. Picador: London.

15 Becoming a reflective learner

This chapter covers:

- reflection as a process of learning;
- models of reflection;
- strategies for developing reflective thinking;
- the context of reflective learning

Hearing the word **reflection** most people automatically think of seeing themselves in a mirror or a pool of still water. Either image means that there is something about yourself that is being played back to you; a form of feedback telling you something about the immediate situation. In the literature this is sometimes called **spective** reflection. A photograph or videofilm will do the same thing but will give you an image of your reflection set in a context in the past, so it is **retrospective**. Likewise a film or a brochure that you see about a place that you plan to visit will also enable you to imagine and reflect on what you might expect to find. Usually you will slot these thoughts into those from other past experiences so that you can interpret them and make sense of them. This is called **prospective** reflection. So you see that you can reflect in the past, the present, and in the future in order to get feedback, and once you have feedback you may wish to do something about what you find out. Just as we have illustrated with visual images and thoughts, so you can reflect like this during your fieldwork placement.

REFLECTION AND LEARNING

According to the educator Professor David Boud (personal communication, May 1994) effective learning will not occur unless you reflect. To do this you must arrest a particular moment in time, ponder over it, go back through it and only then will you gain new insights into different aspects of that situation. According to Kolb (1984) reflecting is an essential element of learning. This is shown through an experiential learning cycle illustrated in Figure 15.1 If you follow this cycle in a clockwise direction you will see that after having had an experience you have to reflect on what you saw or did by reviewing the whole situation in your mind. This may be assisted by looking at it on film, or by discussing it with others. You might then think abstractly about the event for a while. You might seek advice or further information, but eventually you will probably come up with ideas for approaching the situation differently next time. You will then try out your ideas to see if they are effective. You thus complete the learning cycle and start over again with a view to refining your actions. This is an ongoing process so you will never achieve perfection. You will always find other ways of doing things based on your learning from previous experiences.

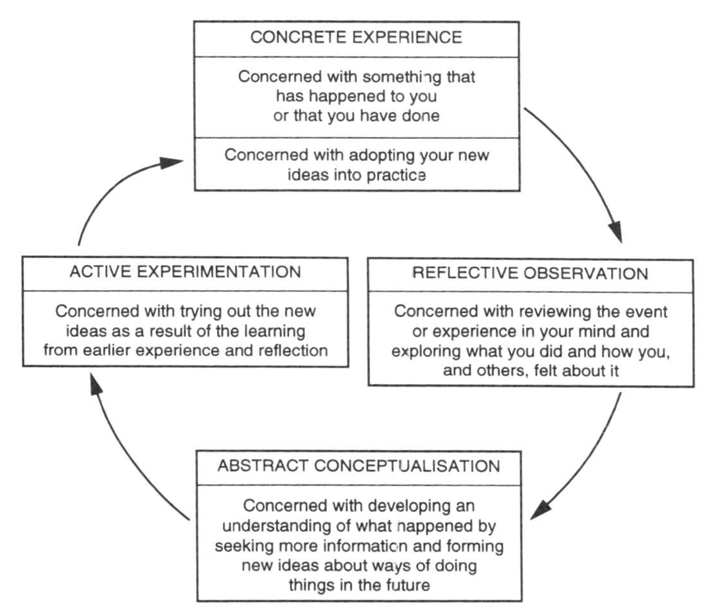

Figure 15.1 Kolb's Learning Cycle

LEVELS OF REFLECTING

In the last chapter we suggested that your clinical reasoning abilities could expand in both breadth and depth. Similarly, your reflective abilities can deepen. According to Van Manen (1977) there are three levels of reflection. The first and most straightforward is concerned with your performance reaching your desired outcomes or objectives. Secondly, you can reflect on any assumptions that you have made in order to see the consequences of different actions. Thirdly, in the highest order, you can reflect on and examine human concerns such as equity and justice. So when you reflect, try to be conscious of, and consider these different levels.

Durgahee (1995) identified three different levels, the macro, the meso, and the micro level. At the macro level, accurate recall of the place, time and people involved in an incident is expected. At the meso level, it should be possible to identify the issues, the interactions and the other building blocks which make up the scene. At the micro level there is concern for the feelings and views of the people involved, the coping strategies used, and the body of knowledge that is needed to make sense of the experience. In addition, this level examines whether new understandings and reasonings have developed, and whether any lessons have been learned from the experience. It seeks to identify whether new-found knowledge can be incorporated into practice to develop alternative ways of working.

MODELS OF REFLECTION

Three models of reflecting are presented here. Each of them contains elements of the other although each is distinctive in its own way. Like other things, one model may appeal to your particular way of learning and working, or it might be more applicable to the setting you are in or to the time you have available to reflect. Each of the authors developed their model at about the same time in the 1980s but the work developed independently in three different countries: Australia, North America, and the UK.

1. The Boud and Walker model

This model from Australia (Boud and Walker, 1991) is presented first as it is the broadest in scope, covering reflection before, during and after an event. It was designed to facilitate both educators' and students' learning and is illustrated in Figure 15.2. The model was developed through its authors' own reflective thinking. An original model designed in 1985 was purely retrospective. This is the part shown in the section on the extreme right-hand side of the model. Not satisfied with this, and after much consultation and deliberation, the present model was formulated as a development from the original. You can see that it contains all three elements of forward, immediate, and retrospective reflection. This model also presents a formula to follow for fieldwork. The first stage could be used for the briefing sessions held at university before your placement starts. The second stage could form the basis of a reflective discussion with your fieldwork educator and academic lecturers during a visit to the fieldwork placement or even be used by yourself in the actual therapeutic session. The last stage could form the outline for the de-briefing sessions once you have finished the placement. You might also use these outlines as a guide to an academic piece of work.

Let us look in more detail at each stage. Try to imagine where you are going on placement, draw on the information given in other chapters in this book and think about your own previous experience.

Preparatory stage

This focuses on three different areas for reflection. Firstly, you should reflect on yourself and have a conversation with yourself. Think about and write down all the

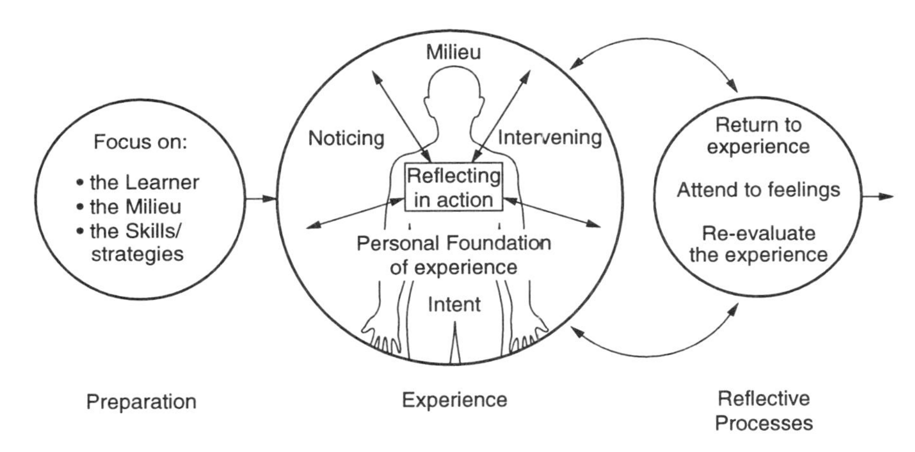

Figure 15.2 Reflection: Boud and Walker's model
Reprinted with permission from Professor David Boud, University of Technology, Sydney, Australia, 1994.
Source: Boud, D and Walker, D. (1990) Making the most of experience. *Studies in Continuing Education,* **12**(2), 67

things that concern you, both in relation to how you are feeling about the placement and your hopes and aims for it. Identify your 'intent' for the placement (see Chapter 9) and be honest about your reasons for going to that particular setting. Remember to note what you are taking to the situation as well as what you want from it.

Secondly, think about what you know already about the placement setting. The first reasoning exercise in Chapter 14 will help you form this future picture and it will show you where the gaps are in your knowledge. Ask yourself, 'what are the rules of the game?' Think about the things that might constrain your learning and what learning opportunities the placement might provide.

Lastly, think ahead about the sort of knowledge and skills you will need for the placement. Do not confine yourself purely to therapeutic skills but think about personal, interpersonal, and managerial skills as well. Follow suggestions given in Chapter 8 for preparing for fieldwork and look back at Chapter 10 for formulating a learning contract. You might want to practise skills or make a videotape to review with a friend. This reflective preparation will help you learn and to feel more confident about the placement so that you can achieve more from it.

Experience stage

Notice that all the stages in this model are bound by a thick outer circle which signifies the context you are in. You should repeat these exercises for each placement as each place is unique.

Let us look at your 'personal foundation of experience'. According to Boud and Walker (1991) it is a folly to underestimate the importance of the knowledge and experience which you bring to a placement. In other chapters we have talked about knowledge gained from personal experience, watching television programmes, reading books or other informal mechanisms. This is referred to in the literature as non-propositional knowledge. The following case story illustrates this.

Case story
While visiting a student on her first fieldwork placement a university lecturer asked the student about an elderly client with rheumatoid arthritis with whom she was working. The student almost recited the procedures she had followed and what had happened during sessions. At no time did the tutor get a sense of the woman as a person so she changed her line of questioning. She asked about the client using a narrative form of reasoning (described in Chapter 14). The student then started describing the 'person' as if she were a neighbour or family member. She also disclosed that her brother had suffered from the same condition for most of his life and she explained the difficulties her family had experienced in coping with this. Suddenly, there was a different picture in front of them. The student had brought all her personal skills and her personal experience into the picture which had changed as a result. This student had a tremendous 'personal foundation of experience' on which to draw, and it is this experience that needs to be elicited by academic and fieldwork educators to assist the student's learning (McKay and Ryan, 1995).

The other construct that requires reflection is your 'intent'. As we have said before, your intent influences your approach to the placement, but if this is at variance with that of others who have planned your programme, a mismatch can result and give rise to counter-productive, disruptive or negative behaviours. Boud and Walker (1991) state that the:

> recognition of learners' intent means that it is rarely possible to set up experiential learning events without either a good understanding of the nature of the participants, or at least the opportunity for participants to influence, in ways meaningful to themselves, the nature of the activity (p. 5).

Reflecting-in-action, as the term suggests, is the ability to reflect while you are actually in the middle of doing something. It is really an extension and refinement of the expression 'thinking on your feet' but it is not quite the same. Rather than just thinking quickly about what to do next, it is more about becoming acutely aware of the situation as if you were both a player in the field and an observer standing outside the arena. This acuteness and awareness of the situation is termed by Boud and Walker as **noticing and intervening**. When you become more critically aware of what is happening in and around you, not only do you notice the actions of the people you see, but you also notice details such as the positions where they stand, the tone of their voice, what they actually say, what they look like and their reactions to events. All this information is absorbed in minute detail as your senses are heightened and alerted to events as they occur. You also become more expert at noting the chronology of events. In essence you are **noticing** events that are relevant to you and your learning, and you will remember them. **Intervening** is trying to visualize how things could be done in a different way. To do this you actually need to break your train of thought by doing something different so that new ideas can develop freely. This is illustrated in the following case story.

Case story
What do you do when things are not going as you planned? Mrs M. was born in Columbia, South America. She had only recently come to live in the USA and she only spoke Spanish although her teenage daughter spoke English. Unfortunately she suffered a stroke (a left CVA) so she was unable to use her right side functionally. She arrived in the clinic accompanied by her daughter and she was seen by an occupational therapist.

On the referral form the need for a translator had not been mentioned and therefore no-one was present. The therapist had an intuitive feeling that if she sent Mrs M. away she would not come back for further work. She decided to continue and to ask for a translator on the following occasion. From the information already on the referral, from questions to the client's daughter and by eliciting a 'Yes' or 'No' response from Mrs M., the therapist started putting the picture together about what had happened and about what functional difficulties were present. She discovered how much the ability to cook was important to Mrs M's perceived role as wife and mother to her family. Suddenly, Mrs M. became upset. Using reflection-in-action, and by noticing and then intervening, the therapist decided to change the whole scenario. She stopped the interview and took Mrs M. to the centre's kitchen where she started to discuss cooking ranges, utensils, and ingredients. Mrs M. became first interested in, and then enthusiastic about, a programme that she could suddenly envisage happening with this therapist. She left the department with more hope for the future and she came back for the following sessions. The translator was there the next time enabling discussion and practical work to be continued. It was only by 'noticing and intervening' that this particular client was not lost to therapy.

Retrospective reflection

This final stage is inextricably bound up with the last phase. You can see this from the diagram and the double headed arrows between the two sections. There seem to be three clusters of activities in retrospective reflection.

Returning to the exercise
The first activity is to return to the experience. This is not as easy as you would imagine. You need to be able to recall and recapture the experience in as much richness and detail as possible. You should bring into your mind all the things that you noticed, and then search your memory for other hidden perceptions. Your memory

can blur unless you train it to be precise. Often you only remember the things you want to. Try to take a snapshot and look at the experience in your mind.

Attending to feelings

Secondly, you need to attend to your feelings which, according to Boud (personal communication, May 1994) can be on two levels. The immediate feeling relates to your own reactions to the event. A more subtle and more difficult feeling to elicit relates to self-awareness, how you reacted, and how you came across to others who were present. Boud believes that you need to re-experience the event and to pay particular attention to the negative feelings that get in the way. These cause blocks which wipe other things out. Once these negative feelings are dealt with you will gain confidence and will be able to move forward to new situations with improved ability and heightened awareness.

Re-evaluating the experience

Thirdly you must re-evaluate the experience. You must make plans to incorporate your new awareness and learning into a similar situation next time. Inevitably you will realize that the situation can never actually be the same because people, time and events change, but you can usefully put your reflections into practice and try again another way. This would be akin to the **active experimentation** phase of Kolb's Learning Cycle. The circle is now complete.

Boud and Walker continue to reflect on and research their thinking in this area and it is likely to evolve in the future.

2. The work of Schon

Professor Donald Schon works at the Massachusetts Institute of Technology (MIT) in North America. His books (Schon, 1983; 1987) on reflection were among the first to be published. Much of his research was done with people in different professions. A wide range of experience was examined to see how reflection might help learning and how becoming a reflective learner might benefit both the person and the profession. Schon explored how expertise develops and identified the stages involved. Although Schon's work is not the focus of this section a summary might help you to put his work on reflection into perspective. Schon's ideas are outlined in Table 15.1.

You can see from the table that reflecting and reasoning development are inextricably intertwined. Schon believes that the process starts with **individual actions or events** set in the larger context of therapy. The ability to understand and to know what you are doing in any situation, coupled with the ability to reflect on this knowing, should enable you to become reflective in action. As you progress through an area of your fieldwork experience using these principles, you gradually see the larger picture of practice, but only within that particular setting. Once this larger picture develops you should be able to reflect on a similar area of practice in other settings and to reflect on interventions overall.

Table 15.1 Process of Schon's development of expertise

Knowing in action + Reflecting on knowing in action	
Reflecting in action	
Developing clinical reasoning	Increased **specialized knowledge** becomes **knowing in practice**. The therapist becomes a **researcher** in his or her own practice, seeking to improve skills and knowledge
	Reflecting on practice enhances interventions
Clinical reasoning in action	**Develops the ability and confidence to criticize initial understanding of a problem and construct a new description**
	UNFORESEEN PROBLEMS/ROADBLOCKS
	Examines personal values and knowledge to see where the defect is, and then changes practice.

Source: adapted from Schon, D. (1983) *The Reflective Practitioner: How Professionals Think in Action*. Basic Books, New York.

Building up experience is a gradual process. As you can see, if you are expected to work through the reflective process in each placement you need to start developing these reflective abilities right away. Reflection should be integral to your sessions with your fieldwork educator. If you examine Schon's thinking in more detail you will see that, by the last stage, you are reflecting at the deeper levels advocated by Van Manen (1977). Use these models and tables as frameworks through which to work with your fieldwork educator.

Schon's ways of reflecting-in-action

Schon's work suggests how you can actually develop reflective abilities during the course of your learning on placement. He believes that reflection should initially develop in safe environments where mistakes are tolerated. You can then reflect and discuss the decisions that were made. For instance, Schon advocates clinical practicums led by the fieldwork educator. Practicums normally involve a client, the fieldwork educator and one or more students. They can be held in the academic setting or in safe environments at the placement. Although simulated clients can be used (played by staff or actors who have been carefully briefed) the best learning occurs when a client co-operates and participates with the therapist in an actual session.

These teaching methods can be likened to coaching. They should not, however, be confused with role play which is different. The educator facilitates the process and students join in with differing levels of participation. Schon offers three methods which are presented here in order of difficulty. Each may suit a particular way

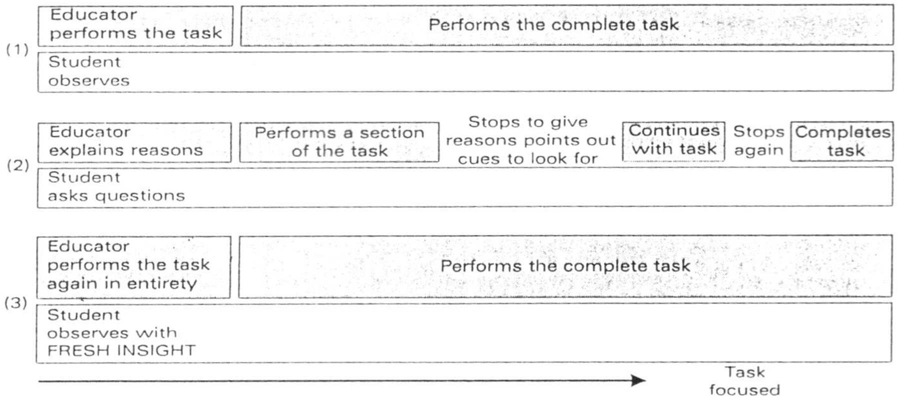

(1)
Educator performs the task | Performs the complete task
Student observes

(2)
Educator explains reasons | Performs a section of the task | Stops to give reasons points out cues to look for | Continues with task | Stops again | Completes task
Student asks questions

(3)
Educator performs the task again in entirety | Performs the complete task
Student observes with FRESH INSIGHT

Task focused

Figure 15.3 Follow Me

Source: adapted from Schon, D. (1987) *Educating the Reflective Practitioner,* Jossey–Bass, San Francisco.

of learning or a particular practice more than the others. Each will contribute to learning in a different way. It is helpful to visualize each method by looking at the relevant diagram.

'Follow Me'

From the title you can see that the fieldwork educator takes the leading role and the student remains more passive in action, although not in perception.

In 'Follow Me' an aspect of practice is chosen by you and your educator. The educator goes through the entire procedure without stopping. You view the performance as if watching television. In watching you will notice certain points, probably those that make sense to you or that tie in with previous experiences. Next the performance is repeated but this time the educator breaks at certain points to make you aware of particular factors that are important or to give you reasons for working in that way. You may be prompted to look at particular features. Signs, symptoms and reactions may be explained. You can enhance your learning in this situation by drawing on theory from your work at university or from personal knowledge. The rehearsal can happen several times depending on the complexity of the procedure. Lastly, the educator repeats the whole performance again without stopping so that you can observe it with new understanding. This method lends itself to being videotaped as a resource for the department and to be watched later. The presentation does not, therefore, always have to be live.

Joint experimentation

This method is more participatory for both student and educator. It can be adapted in different ways depending on what needs to be learnt. It is illustrated in Figure 15.4.

Once again the educator is the prime player. Unlike the last method where you watch the whole performance first, the educator starts the procedure but stops after

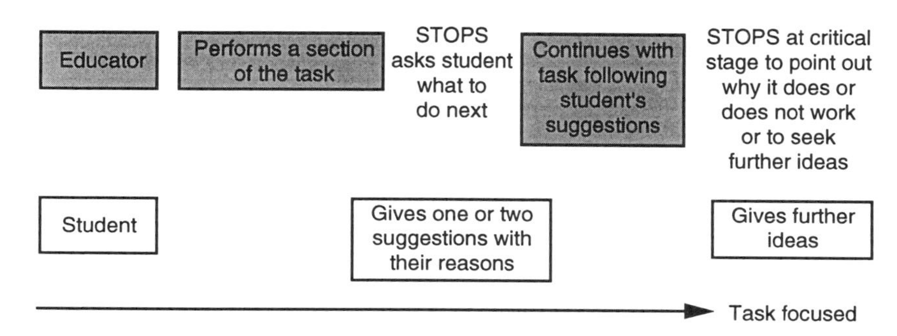

Figure 15.4 Joint experimentation

Source: adapted from Schon, D. (1987) *Educating the Reflective Practitioner,* Jossey–Bass, San Francisco.

a time and asks you what you would do next. You identify options you think might be possible and explain the reasons for your choice. Depending on your reply, the educator proceeds with one avenue of action until either it does not succeed or it leads to the next point. If it does not succeed, the action has at least demonstrated the difficulties that can arise and the things to be aware of and possibly avoid in the future. Learning often emanates from things that go wrong. But here the action is taking place in a safe environment and the educator knows what is possible and what is unsafe. By using this method, not only are actions being demonstrated and explained to you, but your reasoning skills are also being developed. The consequences of your actions thus become apparent.

Hall of mirrors

This method introduces something completely different. You will see that it utilizes many of the deeper points about reflection mentioned earlier in this chapter. For instance it draws on the second and third levels of reflection suggested by Van Manen or else it incorporates some of the points from the final stage of the Boud and Walker model. It is as if you were both looking into a mirror and talking to yourself and to someone else about what you see. This is illustrated in Figure 15.5.

In this method both you and the educator work together much more. You can either both participate in the action, or one or other of you could try something out. After the action you come to a complete stop, as if taking 'time-out'. You then discuss the situation, asking questions such as: 'how does this make me feel?' or 'what difficulties am I experiencing?' As in the diagram, you continue then stop again to discuss another point and reflect. This method not only incorporates the actual performance but it allows individual ideas, and reflections about the situation and about personal reactions to be expressed.

Fish, Twinn and Purr: Strands of Reflection

Fish, Twinn, and Purr (1991) have been developing reflective ways of learning in the UK working in teacher and health visitor education. Their method concentrates more on the retrospective elements of reflection but if followed in entirety, goes into

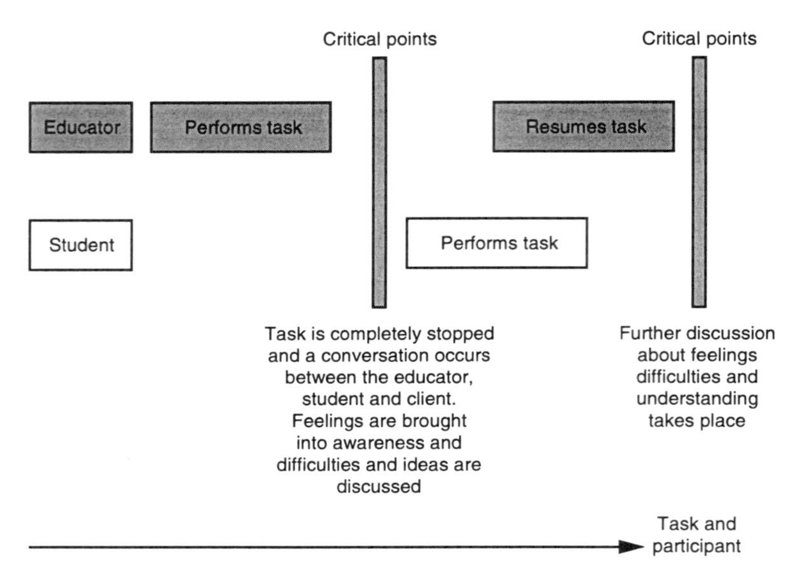

Figure 15.5 Hall of mirrors

Source: adapted from Schon, D. (1987) *Educating the Reflective Practitioner,* Jossey–Bass, San Francisco.

the deep realms of reflection which we mentioned previously. Four Strands of Reflection form this way of learning. Taken together they provide a holistic means of reflecting on practice. All strands include both the cognitive and the affective responses of the person. We can work our way through these strands one by one keeping in mind some of the other aspects of reflection described earlier in this chapter so as to see links as well as gaps, and benefits as well as drawbacks.

The Factual Strand draws mainly on procedural knowledge which is akin to Fleming's (1991) procedural track in clinical reasoning (Chapter 14). It is essentially descriptive and is concerned with the story, including all the chronological events and how the learner felt and reacted to them. When you prepare this strand you must describe it as if you were actually in the scene yourself. Follow this sequence: set the scene, tell the story, pin point any critical incidents, and identify any views, feelings and intentions implicit within the reconstructed practice. Then say what should happen the next time.

The Retrospective Strand is there to develop a personal holistic theory and to critique the entire piece of practice, drawing on the section above. Here you must look back over the experience as a whole. You search for patterns in what happened, and try to elicit new meanings from them. You look at any new knowledge that you have discovered, examine reasons and motives for what took place and explore any critical incidents, failures or successes. Essentially it means putting together your formal knowledge and your personal feelings, and synthesizing these with the needs of the people and the constraints of the context in which you are working. Through this you will become creative and more sensitive to others' points of view since you must gather information from all participants. You therefore start to take account of a range of perspectives which have to be viewed as a whole.

The Sub-Stratum Strand, as its name suggests, is about uncovering and critically exploring personal theories that underlie a piece of practice. In doing this you need to tie your thinking in with formal theories learnt at university. At this level you will be exploring your assumptions, your beliefs and your values that underpin your way of working. We have asked you to consider many of these things already in different chapters of the book as such an awareness is crucial for your professional development. This strand is meant to encourage tolerance of a range of ideas. Often there are no single right answers for occupational therapists' practice which is complex.

The Connective Strand considers how reflections drawn from the previous three strands can be modified for use in future practice, how they relate to it and the practical implications of using them. In doing this you must consider what you have learned from the whole situation and how your thoughts and actions might be modified from this experience.

Table 15.2 outlines the main points of these four strands.

Time for reflection

One thing you must do is to make time for reflection, it has to become part of your way of working and not something separate. It is not a process that can be rushed but neither is it a process that has to occur at a particular time. Thus you can reflect on your journey to or from placement, or between visits to clients, during lunchbreak or even in the middle of the night! You can even sum up each day with a reflective comment in your diary, not spending more than a few minutes doing it. Although you could just ask yourself simple reflective questions such as, 'what happened? how did I feel? how can I do it differently next time?' it does help to have a model of reflection to follow so that you can aim for those deeper levels and insights.

TOOLS THAT AID REFLECTION

Just as we have looked at different ways of reflecting, so too are there different tools to assist you to become a reflective learner. Some of the main ones are described.

Reflective diaries

Before you start this exercise you must clarify who will be reading any diary you might keep. Will you be writing it just for yourself and using selected extracts from it to produce pieces of written work, or will it be seen in its entirety by your fieldwork educator, other students, or your tutors? It is important to establish this from the beginning to avoid surprises at a later date. You can see that what you write could be influenced by who will read it.

Table 15.2 Strands of Reflection: an overview

FOUR STRANDS OF REFLECTION

1. **The Factual Strand**

Restructuring the practice, and drawing mainly upon procedural knowledge of it.

- Setting the scene
- Telling the story
- Pin-pointing the critical incidents
- Identifying views about future practice

2. **The Retrospective Strand**

Developing a wholist theory about, and a critique of, the entire piece of practice, and drawing mainly on procedural knowledge.

- Main patterns visible
- Overall logic
- Overall aims, intentions, goals
- How others might view the practice
- Knowledge discovered
- Analysis of language
- Reason/motive
- Patterns of critical incidents failures, successes etc.

3. **The Sub-Stratum Strand**

Uncovering and exploring critically the personal theory which underlies the piece of practice, and considering how it relates to, and might be helped by, formal theory. Propositional knowledge.

- Customs, beliefs, rituals etc.
- Basic assumptions
- Emerging beliefs about knowledge
- What theories the learner-practitioner has proceeded upon

4. **The Connective Strand**

Considering how present theory and practice might relate to future theory and practice, drawing mainly upon propositional knowledge.

- What has been learned from this situation as a whole? How has it related to past experiences and how might it relate to future ones?
- How might thought and action be modified for future experiences?
- What implications do these reflections have for future practice?

Source: adapted with permission of the publishers from the text of Fish, D. (1995) *Quality Mentoring for Student Teachers: A Principled Approach to Practice*, David Fulton Publishers, London.

Choose a notebook for your diary, not a ring file. You should have something that you can open with a left and right page. Once you have decided which model of reflection to follow, write down your reflective thoughts on the left hand side of the page only. Continue like this for a while recording all your reflective thoughts, feelings and reactions. Don't forget that the more perspectives through which you examine any situation the more you will gain from this exercise. Sometimes it helps to show someone else your diary half way through your placement so that you can make sure you are writing it in a reflective way and not merely recording facts.

Once you near completion of your placement you should go to the next stage.

First take a different coloured pen and then read the diary through in its entirety so that you get a sense of the whole experience. Then go back through your text and put a ring around any incident both positive and negative that made an impression on you. Using this same coloured pen write on the right hand page opposite your present thoughts. Write about the situation but this time say how things could be different or changed the next time around. Finally, at the end of the diary, sum up all your learning experiences from this placement. Think about the impact some of these things have made on you. Consider whether they have changed your understanding or challenged your values at all. Try to visualize where this knowledge is taking you.

Reflective discussion groups

You could set up a focal group where the main aim is to be reflective. It is important to decide who will be in this group. Group work is part of an occupational therapist's repertoire of skills and so it should not be difficult to do. Decide if you will have expert therapists, or only your peers in the group? Will you facilitate it or will you get someone who is impartial to lead the group? Will the group be an open group so others can join in as time goes by, or will you have a closed group for a certain period of time? These are all decisions that have to be made before you start.

Think about using one of the reflective frameworks as this will help you to stay with the subject matter. You can then decide whether one person each time will present work or whether you will consider more than one experience in a session. Don't forget that the closer you are in time to when the experience took place the more real it will seem when you discuss it. The discussions in these groups could also be videotaped if you are willing for the information to be disclosed later for educational purposes.

Videotaping

Opportunities for using videotapes for reflection are enormous. A video takes you right back into the situation so that you can see the players involved and you do not have to rely on your memory. You can use videotapes in a formative way. The educator can prepare them so that you can watch them alone or in groups. You will begin to understand what to look for, ways of working and you can formulate questions for yourself. An enterprising therapist can make an interactive videotape which stops at critical points and asks you what to do next. You can videotape yourself in practice and review the tape yourself. Like the diary, you can choose difficult situations that you would like to discuss with your educator. Alternatively, the educator can view the tape and choose pieces on which to reflect with you. You can work together taking it in turns to control the tape. You can share your work with your colleagues, your peers, or your academic tutors in order to elicit further ideas and perspectives on practice.

You can use videotapes as a summative exercise. If you tape at the beginning and the end of your placement you can see how your performance has progressed. This can be used as a form of assessment which ties in with your learning contract.

Reflective questions

Many of the tools which we have discussed expect you to use reflective processes for learning. The following is a set of questions which you might use to assist your thinking perhaps when you are writing up your reflections on practice in a diary or log, when you are watching a videotape or when you are thinking back over an experience and discussing it with your fieldwork educator.

Reflective questions

- What was I aiming for when I did that?
- What exactly did I do? How would I describe it precisely?
- Why did I choose that particular action?
- What was I trying to achieve?
- What did I do next?
- What were the reasons for doing that?
- How successful was it?
- What criteria am I using to judge success?
- What alternatives were there?
- Could I have dealt with the situation any better?
- How would I do it differently next time?
- What do I feel about the whole experience?
- How did the client feel about it?
- How do I know the client felt like that?
- What sense can I make of this in the light of my past experience?
- Has this changed the way in which I will do things in the future?

CREATING A REFLECTIVE CONTEXT

For reflection to be used to advantage during fieldwork, much will depend on the kind of experience that your fieldwork educator has had in developing an understanding of, and using reflective skills. As we noted at the beginning of this chapter this work is relatively new and many therapists have not yet been exposed to, or had experience in, reflection themselves.

Look out for papers which emphasize the practical use of reflection. For instance, Cross (1993), a physiotherapist, illustrates ways of using reflective exercises on placement and gives samples of students' work. Durgahee (1995) describes in detail the methods used in a course for nurses on using reflection before, during and after the fieldwork experience. Discuss with your fieldwork educator the differences between evaluation, reflection and record keeping. Decide on which framework of reflection you will use on this placement. Boud (personal communication, May, 1994) however, warns that you must be careful not to follow the framework as if it were a set of instructions or a checklist. There should be considerable space for discussion, and all issues must be addressed in a constructive way. Allow time for responses (this is called 'wait time') so that a person responding to a question also has time to reflect on and consider the issue before answering. You might return to the issue when you have all had time to think and reflect on it. Bear in mind that there are many ways of developing reflection as a crucial skill for practice.

SUMMARY

This chapter has explained how reflection is seen as an essential element of learning. It represents one phase of Kolb's Learning Cycle. Reflection can take place at many different levels to enhance understanding of experience and practice. Various models of reflection are presented including the work of Boud and Walker (1991) who advocate reflection before, during and after an event; Schon's (1983) reflection-in-action and Fish, Twinn and Purr's (1991) Strands of Reflection. A number of different strategies are described which would facilitate reflective practice during fieldwork and help develop and maintain a reflective context for learning.

REFERENCES

Boud, D. and Walker, D. (1991) In the midst of experience: developing a model to aid learners and facilitators. Paper presented at the National Conference on Experiential Learning *Empowerment Through Experiential Learning: Explorations of Good Practice*, University of Surrey, 16–18 July 1991.

Cross, V. (1993) Introducing physiotherapy students to the idea of 'reflective practice'. *Medical Teacher*, **15**(4), 293–307.

Durgahee, T. (1995) Teaching reflection: Problems and prospects in nurse education (submitted to *Nurse Inquiry*, Australia).

Fish, D., Twinn, S. and Purr, B. (1991) *Promoting Reflection: The Supervision of Practice in Health Visiting and Initial Teacher Training*. West London Institute Press, London.

Fleming, M. (1991) The therapist with the three track mind. *American Journal of Occupational Therapy*, **45**, 1007–14.

Kolb, D. A. (1984) *Experiential Learning*. Englewood Cliffs, New York.

McKay, E. and Ryan, S. (1995) Clinical reasoning through story telling: Examining a student's case story on a fieldwork placement. *British Journal of Occupational Therapy*, **58**(6), 234–8.

Schon, D. (1983) *The Reflective Practitioner: How Professionals Think in Action*. Basic Books Inc, New York.

Schon, D. (1987) *Educating the Reflective Practitioner*. Jossey-Bass, San Francisco.

Van Manen, M. (1977) Linking up ways of knowing with ways of being practical. *Curriculum Enquiry*, **6**(3), 205–28.

16 Developing competence

This chapter covers:

- concepts of competence;
- development of competence;
- Dreyfus & Dreyfus' continuum of professional development;
- learning strategies for the development of competence;
- assessment of competence.

No book about fieldwork would be complete without a chapter on the development of competence. After all, we have consistently stressed that fieldwork is considered to be an essential component in professional education through which competence to practise is developed, demonstrated and achieved (College of Occupational Therapists 1993a). But what does competence really mean, how does it develop and how would you know if you had achieved it?

WHAT IS COMPETENCE?

A simple dictionary definition of competence (Chambers 1991) suggests that someone who is competent is 'legally qualified' or 'sufficiently good' to do a job. But this simple definition purports to describe something which is anything but simple, as we shall see.

Guttman *et al.* (1988) suggest that competence is an expression of the norms of effective practice in a given profession, it is what the profession expects of its members. Competence encompasses mastery of skills and an understanding of self and clients. These authors maintain that four elements of competence can be facilitated:

intellectual competence:	understanding what to do, when and with whom
performance competence:	understanding how to act in specific situations
personal competence:	self-understanding and the desire to develop one's professionalism
consequence competence:	the ability to determine the extent to which clients were helped.

Consequence competence could arguably also encompass the ability to predict or make an informed judgement about the potential effectiveness or outcome of a course of action. In this analysis the key characteristic of competence appears to be 'understanding'.

Frum and Opacich (1987) similarly define competence as skills, technique, mastery and an ability to take appropriate action. They also consider, however, that a competent practitioner has other attributes such as emotional awareness, autonomy, identity, respect for individual differences, personal motivation, and an ability to state the purpose and direction of plans, giving due consideration to professional ethics. Some of these are personal qualities, others infer a knowledge base.

The College of Occupational Therapists (1993b) expects a competent practitioner to be critically reflective, proactive, innovative and adaptable, capable of working both independently and as a member of a team against a background of social, technical and health care changes. This also suggests that competence embraces many personal qualities and skills, and not just a knowledge base. Additionally, it suggests that competence is seen in the context of a wider environment to which the practitioner has to relate and constantly adjust.

Competence thus has a legal component which aims to safeguard the public, a professional component which requires practitioners to adopt the characteristics and attitudes of the profession, and a context component which requires fitness for practice with a particular client group, in a particular organization and in a constantly changing, wider social, economic and political climate. So we deduce that competence is dynamic and that the maintenance of competence depends on keeping abreast of changes.

Competence as knowledge, understanding and performance

Another way of viewing competence, which emerges from the literature, is to suggest that competence is essentially about three things – knowledge, understanding and performance.

Knowledge is clearly the knowledge base of the profession, its underpinning facts and theories. Some of this knowledge may be tacit knowledge – things that are known but not readily put into words (Barnett, 1994; Mattingly and Fleming, 1994).

Understanding is a conceptual process backed by reason. It must involve the ability to work with concepts, constructs and ideas and not just facts. It is not readily observable but can be tested in dialogue (Barnett, 1994). It is understanding that helps us to make informed decisions in practice.

Performance is about using knowledge, imagination and creativity. It is about sensing and coping with changing circumstances, dealing with unpredictable situations and engaging in problem-setting and problem-solving. Performance depends partly on the quality of current knowledge but it also depends on the judicious use of self in therapeutic situations.

When we add these dimensions to those already discussed, we conclude that competence is multi-dimensional and not easily definable. We can, however, suggest that competence depends on a practitioner's ability to deal effectively with the past, present and future. For instance, it is crucial for the ongoing development of competence that a practitioner is able to reflect-on-action (Schon, 1988) and learn from past experiences with clients. In the present, practitioners are required to manage concurrently an agreed caseload of clients, taking account of each individual's particular needs and, through reflection-in-action, to respond to changes in a timely fashion. Finally, practitioners must have the vision to take account of clients' future life stories, to consider the potential outcomes of interaction and intervention, and the consequences for clients of any future action they take. The skills required for competent performance are thus directly related to reflection, clinical reasoning and professional judgement, all of which have been discussed in earlier chapters.

THE DEVELOPMENT OF COMPETENCE

Having described the perceived components of competence we now take a more practical look at how competence might develop. Benner (1984) and Dreyfus and Dreyfus (1986) see the development of competence as a continuum which includes the stages: **novice, advanced beginner, competent professional, proficient therapist** and **expert**. Cohn and Czycholl (1992) point out that these stages are not meant to be used as a classification system or as a form of labelling, but are intended to help educators understand professional development. Each of the five stages is described in turn and after each we suggest ways to approach learning which should help develop your competence along this continuum.

Dreyfus and Dreyfus Model of Skill Acquisition

Stage 1: working as a novice

If you are completely new to a situation you will probably find that you:

- are able to recognize facts and features of situations;
- attend to separate pieces of information;
- still need to gain confidence by learning and following rules;
- have great difficulty in applying these rules to specific contexts and you have a tendency to generalize them;
- make analogies.

Learning ideas for stage 1

As a novice you will be able to recognize the general facts needed for practice but there will be gaps in your knowledge. Your fieldwork educator should act as a facilitator and help you to discover these missing facts. You might refer to recent articles or books, or a video related to practice, and then share your observations with others to broaden your views and increase your knowledge base. You might also ask your fieldwork educator for written guidelines for practice. Questionnaires or incomplete handouts to fill in will give you something concrete to work with. Consulting the work of Dr Sacks (1986; 1995) will also provide you with a model for writing detailed accounts about clients. Using such a reference will help you become aware of things to look for and things to notice, and thus will help you consolidate your learning. Talking with clients to discover their story is another strategy for developing understanding and competence.

Stage 2: working as an advanced beginner

If you are working at this stage you will:

- consider additional cues and broaden your views;
- start to relate to the client as an individual;
- recognize behaviour but cannot attach meaning to it;
- not see the entire picture as an experienced therapist would.

Learning ideas for stage 2

It is only when you become a little more familiar with what you are trying to do that you start to humanize practice and relate to the client as an individual. As you broaden your view you will become aware of other factors, such as the reactions and behaviours of clients and other people. Try to look closely at what is happening. Examine how you are behaving with the participants as if you were in their story. At this stage you will benefit from hearing about other therapists' ways of working, and their story or narrative of their practice. You might interview a member of staff who was involved in a client's care. Listening to the story, interacting with the story and voicing your views and theories about what happened will help you to develop your own reasoning skills.

Stage 3: working as a competent professional

Now your abilities are really developing, so at this stage you will:

- see actions at least partially in terms of longer-term goals;
- plan consciously and deliberately;
- still follow routine and standardized procedures but you will know which actions are more important than others;
- still lack flexibility and creativity.

Learning at stage 3

This stage of competence is the climax of rule-guided learning. At this stage you need to continue to learn from others. You should participate in group discussions, reflect with others on your work and continue to examine your practice. You might try making a video of yourself talking through a referral. Consciously slow your thoughts down to give yourself time to search for options for intervention. Look for discrepancies in information, for the things that do not fit together. Try to visualize the situation and form an image of what to expect in practice. Talk aloud in order to develop cohesion about what you do.

Stages 4 and 5: working as a proficient practitioner/expert

We include details of these two stages for information.
If you are a proficient therapist you will:

- see situations holistically rather than as components;
- have a sense of direction and vision;
- be able to deal with unfamiliar situations;
- manage decision-making well;
- modify initial findings as meanings vary and according to the situation.

If you are working as an expert you will:

- no longer rely on rules;
- have an intuitive grasp of situations based on deep tacit knowledge;
- use analytic approaches only when working in new situations or when problems occur;
- have a vision of what is possible based on reflective experience.

Learning at stages 4 and 5
Stages 4 and 5 of Dreyfus and Dreyfus' model only emerge after three to five years of practice experience and as such they do not occur in your undergraduate education. They are presented here to give you something to aim for. It is expected that, once qualified, you will continue to strive for proficiency and expertise in practice.

LEVELS OF COMPETENCE

It is worth noting that there are many levels of competence. Competence, albeit at a minimum level, is required for state registration. Hopefully, however you will be striving for at least an optimum level of competence before you qualify, and some of you will achieve more. Additionally, as a competent practitioner, you should have a commitment to the development of higher levels of competence, that is, mastery and proficiency in skilled performance. If you take no responsibility for continuing your professional development after qualifying you are likely to become incompetent!

Mocellin (1984) noted that competence does not equate with excellence or the ability to do everything. Instead he recognized that there are degrees of sufficiency and adequacy in people. This is pertinent to our discussion about the development of competence. Individuals enter university with different levels of skills and develop at different rates through their course of study. The level of competence attained by each individual on qualification will therefore vary. The minimum standard for safe practice will apply when a judgement is made about an individual's competence to practice as an independent, qualified practitioner.

Attaining professional competence is obviously a requirement for your State Registration and for professional practice with clients, but a judgement about your competence is likely to be a subjective one however well the criteria for judging competence are defined. Ilott (1995) quoted a case in the US Supreme Court where the fieldwork educator's right to make a subjective judgement was upheld given that clinical behaviour was judged against acceptable standards. It is for this reason that the profession places so much emphasis on the education and accreditation of fieldwork educators who ultimately have to make that judgement.

ASSESSING COMPETENCE

In order to judge your competence at qualifying level there needs to be some concept of competence. It is important to know what attributes are required of a competent practitioner so that those who demonstrate them can be recommended for State Registration. As we have shown, competence is about knowledge, understanding and performance. It is also about personal attributes and qualities which are difficult to measure. It is about **how** these qualities are used and **how well** these qualities are used in practice.

Bondy (1983) helps us to think about the assessment of the quality of performance. She analysed the competent performance of nurses and devised a structured system for evaluating competence. This entailed defining performance standards and assessing students in terms of how **safely, accurately, efficiently and effectively** they performed their duties, the **manner** in which they were performed (the demeanour of the practitioner when carrying out the performance standard) and how much **assistance** was required. It was noted, however, that seeking and using assistance appropriately was considered acceptable behaviour. Bondy's model of assessment was used as a basis for the development of a model for assessing the competence of Occupational Therapy students (Alsop 1993).

A developmental model in fieldwork

Alsop's (1993) model, shown in Figure 16.1, requires students on fieldwork to focus on developing competence in five core elements: safe practice, professional standards and behaviour, client-centred care, Occupational Therapy process and professional relationships. Once the student is judged to be performing at a competent level, attention can be paid to a further five skills: communication, reflective practice, personal and work management and integration of theory and practice. It is suggested that the latter set of skills develops over time and, for some, competence in these elements will only be demonstrated after qualification. A pass mark in these further skills is not required for professional qualification whereas a pass in the five core elements is essential. By giving weighting to the core elements, weaker students can prioritize their learning to concentrate on developing the skills said to be essential for competent practice at the most basic level.

Incompetence

Some fieldwork evaluation forms have performance criteria against which students are assessed. If the student meets the appropriate performance criteria he or she is considered to be practising competently. Where there is doubt, the written criteria for failing a student serve as a guide for decision-making. They are indicators that competence has not been demonstrated. This is not to say necessarily that a student is incompetent, although in a small proportion of cases that might be so, it is just

First level	Dependent	Directed	Assisted	Supervised	Self-directed		
Higher level	Dependent	Dependent	Directed	Assisted	Supervised	Self-directed	
1	Unsafe practice *or*	Safe practice	Safe practice	Safe practice	Safe practice	Safe practice	1
2	Unprofessional behaviour	Professional behaviour *but*	Professional behaviour	Professional behaviour	Professional behaviour	Professional behaviour	2
Core Skill Area		*underdeveloped:*					
3		Client-centred care	Client-centred care	Client-centred care	Client-centred care	Client-centred care	3
4		OT process *or*	OT process	OT process	OT process	OT process	4
5		Professional relationships	Professional relationships	Professional relationships	Professional relationships	Professional relationships	5
6				Communication	Communication	Communication	6
7				Reflective practice	Reflective practice	Reflective practice	7
8					Personal management	Personal management	8
9					Work management	Work management	9
10						Integration of theory and practice	10

Figure 16.1 Developmental model of skill acquisition
Reprinted with permission

Source: Alsop, A. (1993) The developmental model of skill acquisition in fieldwork, *British Journal of Occupational Therapy*, **56**(1), 7–12

that competence has yet to be developed and demonstrated. The onus is always on the student to demonstrate competent behaviour, it is not the responsibility of the fieldwork educator to assume competence in the absence of evidence. It is expected that when a judgement to fail a student is made, the fieldwork educator can specify particular incidents or examples from the student's work to justify the decision.

A checklist for evaluating competence

Self-assessment is a very important skill to develop for professional practice. To help you to evaluate your own performance and level of competence in fieldwork, we provide a schedule of questions which you might ask yourself. Some of the questions shown in Table 16.1 are derived from Bondy's model for evaluating clinical performance.

PROFESSIONALISM AS A PRACTICAL ART

The schedule of questions might provide a useful structure to aid reflection and skill development, but does not provide a complete picture of competence. Throughout

Table 16.1 Schedule of questions to ask after completion of a task: facilitating personal competence

Professional knowledge and skill
1 Did I have the knowledge needed for the task?
2 Did I have the technical skills for the task?

Proficiency
3 Did I perform safely and take the necessary safety precautions?
4 Did I put anyone at risk?
5 Did I perform accurately?
6 Did I use resources effectively?
(energy, materials, equipment)
7 Did I complete the task within a reasonable timescale?
8 Did I achieve my intended purpose?

Interpersonal skill
9 Did I act in an appropriate manner?
(was my communication and demeanour professional; did I show sensitivity to others?)

Assistance
10 How much assistance did I need?
11 To what extent did I make independent professional judgements?

Reasoning and judgement
12 Could I discuss the reasoning for my judgements and decisions?
13 Would I do anything different next time?
14 Do I need to develop my knowledge base or level of skill?
15 To what extent have I attained mastery in this aspect of the work?

the book we have been encouraging you to develop skills of the **practical artist** (Fish *et al.*, 1991) instead of relying on technical rational methods of operating. We need to consider how the characteristics of the two models fit with our understanding of competence.

We have already said that technical rational methods use rules and structures and provide a framework in which to work, but that these can also set boundaries for practice which can sometimes be unhelpful and restrictive. For the technician, competent performance is about acting routinely and by prescription. As a contrast, the practical artist exercises judgement about the use of rules in his or her practice, acts creatively and develops ways of working to meet changing needs and circumstances. Knowledge is treated as a temporary feature and is constantly revised in the light of new experience and developments. Competence embraces creativity rather than rigidity in practice. Over time, obsolete theories are rejected and new theories are integrated into practice. This reinforces our assertion that competence is transient and not easily definable.

COMPETENCE AND CONTINUING PROFESSIONAL DEVELOPMENT

Given that competence is dynamic, and that the demands of practice and the practice environment are constantly changing, continuing professional development is essential. It is essential on two counts, firstly because it is necessary for a practitioner to maintain competence which means keeping up to date with changes and making sure that he or she is acquainted with new knowledge and theories in the relevant field of practice, and secondly so that personal expertise develops beyond a basic level of competence. These are professional expectations (College of Occupational Therapists, 1995) and each practioner has a responsibility to take steps to update knowledge and develop skills through whatever means seem appropriate.

The following is taken from the American *Guide to Fieldwork Education* (updated 1994):

> Professional competence is attained through the process of self-directed learning and contributes to the development of clinical reasoning. It is the professional and ethical responsibility of each practitioner to continue his or her own professional growth through varied learning opportunities. Such opportunities may include formal continuing education programs, published materials, and collegial consultation [participating in formal discussion with colleagues]. Consultation or a formal mentoring arrangement with content specialists may provide the entry-level practitioner with a more in-depth learning strategy. A competent practitioner is one who:
>
> - identifies needs;
> - identifies resources;
> - selects appropriate options;
> - implements professional competence plans (p. 265).

Professional growth will only occur if it is actively sought. This is borne out by Ryan's (1990) study. She found evidence to suggest that some therapists with several years of exerience were still working in a technical mode and that they had not grown professionally or moved to higher levels of competence and reasoning.

As a final point, two things are worth reiterating, firstly, that ongoing learning is essential to the maintenance of competence and secondly, that you are learning to be a **master** or **expert** in Occupational Therapy and not a 'jack of all trades'. Three words therefore sum up the skills needed for being able to move beyond competence: reflecting, enquiring and creating. These activities underpin both creative professional practice and academically rigorous learning (Lester, 1995).

SUMMARY

This chapter has explored the meaning of competence. Competence is said to embrace elements of intellectual, performance, personal and consequence competence and to have legal, professional and context components. Knowledge, understanding and performance are factors involved in competent practice. A qualifying practitioner may operate at one of several levels of competence. An understanding of the stages of competence development from novice to expert can help in determining learning needs. The assessment of competence is a subjective matter. Self-assessment enables the student to participate actively and define strengths, limitations and needs. Explicit statements which define incompetent as well as competent performance can assist fieldwork educators to assess whether a student has failed or passed the fieldwork placement. The maintenance of competence depends on continuing professional development using skills of reflection, enquiry and creativity.

REFERENCES

Alsop, A. (1993) The developmental model of skill acquisition in fieldwork. *British Journal of Occupational Therapy*, **56**(1), 7–12.

Barnett, R. (1994) *The Limits of Competence, Knowledge, Higher Education and Society*. The Society for Research into Higher Education and Open University Press, Buckingham.

Benner, P. (1984) *From Novice to Expert*. Addison-Wesley, Reading, MA.

Bondy, K. N. (1983) Criterion-referenced definitions for rating scales in clinical evaluation. *Journal of Nursing Education*, **22**(9), 376–82.

Chambers Concise Dictionary (1991) W & R Chambers, Edinburgh.

Cohn, E. and Czycholl, C. (1992) Facilitating a foundation for clinical reasoning. In E. Crepeau and T. LaGarde, *Self-Paced Instruction for Clinical Education and Supervision (SPICES)*. The American Occupational Therapy Association, Inc, MD.

College of Occupational Therapists (1993a) *Guidelines for Assuring the Quality of the Fieldwork Education of Occupational Therapy Students*. SPP 165, College of Occupational Therapists, London.

College of Occupational Therapists (1993b) *Curriculum Framework for Occupational Therapy*. SPP161, College of Occupational Therapists, London.

College of Occupational Therapists (1995) *Code of Ethics and Professional Conduct for Occupational Therapists*. College of Occupational Therapists, London.

Dreyfus, H. and Dreyfus, S. (1986) *Mind over Machine*. The Free Press, Macmillan, New York.

Eraut, M. (1989) Initial Teacher Training and the NVQ Model. In J. Burke (ed.), *Competency Based Education and Training,* The Falmer Press, London.

Eraut, M (1994) *Developing Professional Knowledge and Competence*. Falmer Press, London.

Fish, D., Twinn, S. and Purr, B. (1991) *Promoting Reflection: The Supervision of Practice in Health Visiting and Initial Teacher Training*. West London Institute Press, London.

Frum, D. and Opacich, K (1987) *Supervision: Development of Therapeutic Competence*. The American Occupational Therapy Association, Inc. MD.

Guide to Fieldwork Education (1994) American Occupational Therapy Association Inc. Bethesda, MD.

Guttman, E., Eisikovits, Z. and Maluccio, A. N. (1988) Enriching Social Work supervision from the competence perspective. *Journal of Social Work Education*, Fall, no. 3, 278–88.

Ilott, I. (1995) To fail or not to fail? a course for fieldwork educators. *American Journal of Occupational Therapy*, **49**(3), 250–5.

Lester , S. (1995) Beyond knowledge and competence: towards a framework for professional education. *Capability*, **1**(3), 44–52.

Mattingly, C. and Fleming, M. H. (1994) *Clinical Reasoning: Forms of Inquiry in a Therapeutic Practice*. F.A. Davis Company, Philadelphia.

Mocellin, G. (1984) Adaptation, coping or competence? theoretical choices and professional decisions in occupational therapy. In Proceedings of the Australian Association of Occupational Therapists 13th Federal Conference, Perth. Australian Occupational Therapy Association, Vol. 2.

Raven, J. (1995) The universities, the development of competence and public policy. *Capability*, **1**(3), 3–6.

Ryan, S. (1990) *Clinical Reasoning: A Descriptive Study Comparing Novice and Experienced Occupational Therapists*. Unpublished master's thesis, Columbia University, New York.

Sacks, O. (1986) *The Man who Mistook his Wife for a Hat*. Pan Books, London.

Sacks, O. (1995) *An Anthropologist on Mars*. Picador, London.

Schon, D. (1988) From technical rationality to reflection in action. In J. Dowie and A. Elstein (eds), *Professional Judgement: a Reader in Clinical Decision Making*. Cambridge University Press, Cambridge.

Being assessed

17

This chapter covers:

- the purpose of assessment;
- the process of assessment;
- the grading of performance.

All too often the concept of assessment provokes feelings of anxiety amongst students who are quick to identify the negative, rather than the positive, aspects of the assessment process. There seems to be an overriding concern that behaviour and performance during fieldwork education will be observed every minute of the day and that putting a foot wrong will have a detrimental effect on the final evaluation of practice. So let us start by dispelling a few myths so that assessment and evaluation of practice can be seen in a positive light. The first thing to do is to explore the purpose of assessment.

PURPOSE OF ASSESSMENT

Primarily an assessment is to provide evidence to a university that a student has followed a course of study, understood its content, mastered its objectives and can demonstrate mastery on his or her own (Nuttall and Barnes, 1981). Students in programmes in the UK leading to Occupational Therapy qualification must also be assessed to meet professional and legal requirements for State Registration. The assessment process aims to establish whether competence has been achieved. Successful performance wins a licence for the individual to practise Occupational Therapy within society. Quite reasonably, therefore, the public has a right to expect that an individual's mastery or competence is confirmed through an assessment process before the individual is allowed to practise on his or her own. The purpose of assessment here is to maintain professional standards and through that to safeguard the public.

The reality, however, is that no student can be expected to master every objective and not every objective can necessarily be addressed through formal assessment. Pring (1991, cited in Brown and Knight, 1994) points out that competence involves 'expert behaviour' which is not bound by rules and not readily prescribed. This suggests that professional performance cannot exclusively be assessed as the application of knowledge and skills in practice against fixed criteria on an assessment schedule. It suggests that professional performance has a further quality or dimension which ought to be subject to assessment but which cannot be defined in the form of objectives. The **purpose** of assessment nevertheless must be to determine whether the individual can demonstrate sufficient expert behaviour to be considered competent to practise.

Let us take purpose a stage further. The assessment process can also provide for diagnosis (Rowntree, 1987) as a mechanism for identifying a student's strengths and limitations. This diagnosis can be beneficial. When strengths are identified there is usually positive feedback which serves as a motivating factor for future performance. When limitations and needs are identified the student can be helped to work on deficits and develop the competence needed for practice. But who should take responsibility for diagnosing strengths and needs?

Self-assessment to identify strengths and needs

Boud (1990) argues for self-assessment. Learning, he says, is an active endeavour where only the learner can implement decisions that affect his or her learning. The student must therefore be involved in identifying strengths and needs. Being involved in assessing your own work provides you with a formal opportunity to critique your performance and diagnose your own strengths and limitations. You can then direct your attention to improving those aspects of your performance which are not reaching the required standard. It can focus your mind so that you can build on your strengths and modify what you do in order to pay more attention to deficits in skills and weaker areas of practice. We shall see in a moment how responsibilities are actually shared between the fieldwork educator and the student, but it seems that assessment and particularly self-assessment, has a facilitative function in your preparation for professional life.

Ongoing assessment can also assist in determining how you are progressing towards meeting short- and longer-term goals. If you have a learning contract you can assess your achievements yourself against the agreed action plan and revise the contract to reflect new needs and goals. The contract can provide a sense of purpose, the assessment can provide a sense of achievement.

THE ASSESSMENT PROCESS

On several occasions in the book we have referred to learning contracts, aims, objectives, goals and learning outcomes. The assessment of practice will involve examining carefully just how well you have approached and addressed the tasks required of you and achieved the set objectives. This will be done through supervision sessions where you will be required to reflect on your performance, and sometimes on the performance of others. If you are using a learning contract, your performance in relation to the agreed action plan will be assessed using whatever mechanism was agreed in the contract.

Both you and your fieldwork educator will be involved in evaluating your work and you will be given feedback which should guide future practice. A final assessment of fieldwork education will be made at the end of the placement which must indicate how well you are performing at that time and in that setting, taking into account the stage you are at in your course.

In placements occurring early in your programme, this may be quite straight forward. The experience may be new to you but the assessment should not be feared. After all, everyone realizes that you are there to learn and this will be reflected in both the process and outcome of the assessment. In later placements there will be more demands made of you and more expectations than in earlier placements. The client group with which you are working may, however, be very new to you and make different demands in terms of using your knowledge and skills. Even though you may be in the final year of your course, everything on a placement may be new to you. In these situations you will be expected to draw on knowledge and previous experiences to help you to work with this client group. You will be expected to apply Occupational Therapy principles and processes in the new situation. You are, after all, learning to practise Occupational Therapy in all sorts of areas and with all sorts of clients.

You may well feel more comfortable with some clients than with others, or in some settings than in others, but the variety of experience is important for your future practice. If you are unhappy or uncomfortable with a particular client group then you should do the best you can. Talk to your fieldwork educator about your difficulties since these might affect your assessment. Your fieldwork educator might be able to suggest some alternative approaches that you might take. All experience can contribute to your learning even if you choose not to practise Occupational Therapy with such a client group when you are qualified.

Making mistakes

Often students feel that their performance on placement must be perfect at all times. This is totally unrealistic. The fieldwork setting is often considered the place where, within reason, you are allowed to make mistakes – so that you can learn from them. Fieldwork education provides a relatively safe and supportive environment for practising new skills and for trying out new ideas. No fieldwork educator will allow clients to be exploited or put at risk for the sake of a student's learning, but most educators will allow some flexibility for students to put their ideas into practice so that they can experience the consequence of their plans and actions. These ideas will obviously need to be carefully thought through and discussed with the fieldwork educator. Debriefing should consider the extent to which the plan and its implementation was a success.

As far as your assessment goes, it is far more important for you to understand what went well in a situation and why, or what went wrong and what you would do differently next time, than just to know that something did go wrong and not be able to explain it. Assessment of your practice should take account of your ability to evaluate your performance and learning and not just the outcome of your actions.

Formative and summative assessment

You may well have heard of the terms **formative** and **summative** assessment in relation to your academic work. The main purpose of formative assessments is to enable learning, whereas the main purpose of summative assessments is to test and confirm the learning that has taken place. Formative assessments do not normally count towards awards whereas summative assessments do. Formative assessments allow for feedback on performance so that performance can be improved and so that personal and professional development can take place. Summative assessments are often completed at the end of a period of study and feedback may or may not be given on performance. So formative assessments and summative assessments perform different functions. Although this is a slightly simplistic way of looking at it, formative assessments help **you** to improve your competence to practise, while summative assessments primarily inform **the university** that you merit the award.

Collaborative assessment

As far as fieldwork is concerned, formative assessments are usually seen as ongoing discussions which take place between you and your fieldwork educator at regular intervals during the placement. This may include a formative assessment as a requirement of the university which is carried out midway through the placement. Formative assessment of your placement can take place collaboratively where both you and your fieldwork educator make separate assessments of your performance in relation to the agreed objectives and then you come together to discuss the outcome.

This collaborative process allows you to assess your strengths and needs and agree them with your fieldwork educator. There may be times when the two of you will have different perceptions about your performance. Often students underestimate their ability and where their strengths lie. The fieldwork educator can provide a different, and often more positive perspective.

Concern often arises, however, when a student thinks that his or her performance is good but the fieldwork educator thinks otherwise. Some students misjudge a situation, but through discussion develop a better understanding of what is required. Some students find it hard to evaluate their own performance and need guidance and practice in reflection and self-evaluation. Other students just do not seem to have insight into their limitations and needs. A skilled fieldwork educator may need to provide fairly structured feedback in this instance so that concerns are pointed out and there is clarity about performance and expectations in the future.

If this happens to you, you would be advised to consider how well you receive and use this feedback and the constructive criticism of your work. However uncomfortable it may be to hear someone else's view of your performance, a positive approach to using this criticism should enable you to become a better practitioner.

The ability to assess one's own performance critically and accurately is a professional skill which needs to be developed. Clearly, qualified professionals must have the ability to assess whether their input to a client's care has been effective, to record their evaluation of a completed case in the client's notes, to contribute effectively to peer review and to participate actively in any more formal appraisal of their own performance as part of a personal development programme.

The fieldwork experience provides the opportunity to practise self-evaluation skills. The ultimate goal is for a student to become a self-disciplined professional who uses self-evaluation as a normal part of everyday practice and who can judge the effectiveness of his or her actions and so learn to improve performance in the future.

Keeping records of supervision

A record of your discussions with your fieldwork educator should be kept in the interests of you both. The summary should be dated, indicate the feedback given, note any improvements in performance, and show how newly identified needs may be addressed.

GRADING OF PERFORMANCE

With a few exceptions, programmes leading to Occupational Therapy qualification in the UK are either ordinary bachelors or honours degrees. Fieldwork education within an ordinary degree programme, and in some honours degree programmes, is normally graded as either fail or pass. Occasionally merit is awarded for exceptional performance where the regulations allow.

Some honours degrees have more complex systems of grading fieldwork because the university awarding the degree expects fieldwork to be assessed in exactly the same way as academic work (Alsop, 1993). A percentage mark has to be determined from the grade awarded for the placement so that the mark can be used in calculating the classification of the degree. In this case there will usually be five bands or grades on the assessment scale to match the classification bands, i.e.

1st class honours

2nd class honours – upper division

2nd class honours – lower division

3rd class honours

fail

The names of the grades for fieldwork which are associated with each of the classification bands are different in each university. Some may use a points scale, others may use an alphabetical range (e.g. A–E). Some may use qualitative statements on a continuum from exceptional performance to fail. All will require some kind of conversion to a percentage for determining the degree classification.

Grading of fieldwork education as a pass or fail is usually fairly straight forward for the fieldwork educator, especially where criteria for failure are clearly defined. If you are awarded a pass, even at the lowest level, you are considered to be competent to practise, albeit at a basic level. The difficulty comes when fieldwork educators are asked to determine which grade beyond the basic competent pass grade should be awarded. There are often three other pass grades to choose from. Awarding a higher grade on the scale should reflect qualitatively better performance and higher achievement than the basic pass grade, but as with any assessment of competence the judgement can be subjective.

When grading performance, fieldwork educators are asked to be honest about a student's level of ability. It is important that they are not driven by a student's desire for a high grade but remain as objective as possible and judge performance against the criteria defined. It is not in your interests for you to be given a false impression of what you can or cannot do. A fair assessment of your performance is what is required. This means that fieldwork educators will not be asked to assess your potential but will be asked to report on your present ability against the set criteria. You may come out with a lower grade than you might have expected, but this is because the mark awarded indicates the minimum level of performance which can be expected of you at another time or in a similar situation (Bondy, 1983). She argues that if only the best aspects of your performance are judged and reflected in the grade, some areas of your performance that would benefit from further teaching or development may be obscured.

Whatever system of grading is used, you need to be sure that you understand it and know what is required of you. If you find yourself in a programme which uses a grading system as part of the degree classification process you would be well advised to look carefully at the requirements for the lowest level and the highest level pass grade to establish what you will be expected to do, and how you will be expected to perform to be awarded those grades. You then have the basis for discussion with your fieldwork educator and you can agree how you might work towards fulfilling the assessment requirements.

One word of warning, do keep in mind that fieldwork is essentially a learning experience and not one where you merely need to pass the assessment or gain a good grade. Most students want to do well during their placement but if you focus only on the requirements for being awarded a high grade, you could miss so many learning opportunities. You are learning to practise Occupational Therapy not just 'to get by' in the placement and it is your responsibility as a developing professional to ensure that you take advantage of the learning opportunities on offer.

Negotiated assessment

Negotiated assessment is used in some programmes. It starts with the process of collaborative assessment but the student and fieldwork educator go on to negotiate and agree a grade to be awarded for the placement. Where there is discrepancy, each offers a rationale for awarding a particular grade. Where no negotiated agreement can be reached, the fieldwork educator has the responsibility for awarding the final grade. The student can note any disagreement so that university staff are aware of the difference in perception.

Half-way report

Some universities require fieldwork educators to complete a report of a student's progress half way through a placement. Whatever the process used to determine progress, some judgement will be made about how the student is performing at this stage of the placement. The report is normally formative but may still serve as a formal procedure for identifying strengths and future needs. At this stage, objectives should be renegotiated to ensure that, in the remaining weeks of the placement, learning needs can be met. A copy of the half-way report is sent to the university, one is kept by the fieldwork educator and one by the student.

The final report

The final evaluation of your practice is the summative assessment which counts towards your degree. The outcome of your performance during fieldwork may be decided through a collaborative or negotiated process, but the fieldwork educator normally has the final responsibility for determining the grade awarded. The grade is recorded on the final report which is then returned to the university. This is the formal record of your performance in the placement. It usually confirms the hours that you have completed as well as the grade you have achieved. It would be normal for both you and your fieldwork educator to keep a copy.

APPEALS AGAINST ASSESSMENT DECISIONS

Appeals procedures governing the assessment of fieldwork education are laid down by the university. They are often the same as for the assessment of any academic work. Although each university will have a different system the two most common grounds for appeal are firstly, that the student's performance in the assessment was adversely affected by illness or other extenuating circumstance which he or she, for valid reasons, was unable or unwilling to divulge prior to the assessment, and secondly, that there is satisfactory evidence that there has been a material administrative error in the way in which the assessment was conducted. No challenge to the grade awarded for fieldwork education is normally allowed. You should acquaint yourself with your own university regulations governing assessments and appeals and note the timespan in which an appeal should be lodged. Appeals procedures do not normally come into effect until after an Examination Board has sat and confirmed the results of an assessment.

If you feel aggrieved in any way about the outcome of your fieldwork experience you should notify the university immediately and set down in writing the comments that you wish to make. Keep the comments factual and quote relevant dates and incidents to support your case. Give the comments to your tutor and keep a copy for yourself. Establish the forum for dealing with your concerns.

AVOIDING FAILURE

If you feel that your fieldwork experience is not going well then it is in your best interests to contact a member of the university staff as soon as possible and outline the difficulties. The half-way report, or feedback during supervision sessions, should have alerted you to problems which need to be addressed. We always say that a final report indicating that a student has failed the placement should be no surprise to the student. This is because he or she will have had relevant feedback earlier in the placement and will have been given the opportunity to remedy problems.

Where there are problems the university may expect you to explore them with your fieldwork educator in the first instance although university staff will arbitrate if requested. If problems are serious, or where there is potential for you failing the placement, your university tutor will expect to be informed at the earliest possible moment. In this way, the problems can be explored together and a plan agreed to give you the opportunity to succeed.

Where failure is anticipated it is important for you to have some clear direction about remedial action which can be taken. You will need help and support to analyse the problem and set priorities in order to work towards a pass grade. You will need to be clear about your responsibilities and the action you must take. It is good practice for an action plan to be put in writing so that it serves as a checklist and guide. You can return to it frequently, upgrading it as necessary to reflect your progress towards achieving identified goals. You should also establish the regularity and nature of supervision that you can expect from your fieldwork educator as you work through the problems, and the nature of support which you can expect from a member of the university staff.

Failing and retaking a fieldwork placement

While it can be upsetting for everyone involved if you fail a placement, sometimes it is actually in your best interests. In the event of a first-time failure you will almost certainly be given an opportunity to retake the assessment in another fieldwork setting. Some students need that extra time to learn about practice and benefit considerably from the additional experience which a further placement offers. Some learning will have taken place even if your experience is graded as a fail. If you do fail, you need to be clear about what you learnt from the experience, what your ongoing needs are and how you are going to address them the next time round. Write these down and use reflective learning principles to see what you need to do differently next time.

One of the most difficult decisions to make is whether to inform the new placement of the fact that you have failed in the previous setting. You should clarify with your course tutor what the new fieldwork educator will be told about your needs. Often it will be left to you to tell your fieldwork educator that you have failed a placement if you wish to do so. It can be in your best interests to tell the staff but you should do it objectively and without criticizing the earlier placement. State what you learnt from the experience and identify your needs in the new setting. While sometimes there are concerns that a fieldwork educator's knowledge of a previous failure may adversely affect the next assessment, most fieldwork educators prefer to work in an atmosphere of honesty and openness.

SUMMARY

This chapter has addressed the process of assessment, including the use of feedback and the grading of performance. Assessment of your fieldwork practice is largely intended to enable you to develop the skills needed for professional work. It should be seen as a positive, constructive process rather than just the outcome of a placement which is summed up in the grade awarded for your performance. Assessment is a process in which you should participate and play an active part because it is a process of learning which contributes to your personal and professional development. Self-assessment and constructive feedback should be seen as positive mechanisms in the assessment process through which you can learn and grow. Even failing a placement can produce positive learning.

REFERENCES

Alsop, A. (1993) The developmental model of skill acquisition in fieldwork. *British Journal of Occupational Therapy*, 56(1), 7–12.

Bondy, K. N. (1983) Criteria-referenced definitions for rating scales in clinical evaluation. *Journal of Nurse Education,* 22(9) 376–82.

Boud, D. (1990) Assessment and the promotion of academic values. *Studies in Higher Education*, 17(2), 185–200.

Nuttall, D. L. and Barnes, P. (1981) *Examinations and Assessment. Contemporary Issues in Education.* Block 4. Open University, Milton Keynes.

Pring, R. (1991) *Competence.* Paper presented to the UCET conference, Oxford. In S. Brown and P. Knight, *Assessing Learners in Higher Education.* Kogan Page, London.

Rowntree, D. (1987) *Assessing Students: How Shall We Know Them?* Kogan Page, London.

18 Evaluating the fieldwork experience

This chapter covers:

- self evaluation of the fieldwork experience;
- informal evaluation with peers;
- formal debriefing at the university.

Evaluation is an integral part of the learning process. It might be thought of as the rounding up of any event or experience which allows for systematic reflection on, and confirmation of, learning and the identification of new goals.

Your fieldwork educator will have evaluated your practice and presented you with a written report at the end of your placement. In the final discussion with your fieldwork educator you will have gained some insights into your strengths and limitations and have been given some constructive advice about your future learning.

You may also have completed a fieldwork evaluation about the placement and presented it to your fieldwork educator. We talked about how you might write and present constructive feedback in Chapter 9.

Two further things should ideally take place at the end of your fieldwork experience. Firstly you should take time alone to think back over the total experience and consider what personal learning has taken place. Secondly you should participate in a debriefing session at your university. You should be guided to consider the relevance of this particular fieldwork experience to your professional education and development. Let us consider each of these in turn.

YOUR EVALUATION OF THE PLACEMENT

Thinking back over the whole experience, and thinking of the experience as a whole, take time to reflect on the questions in Tables 18.1 and 18.2. These address:

1. your preparation for, and participation in, fieldwork;
2. your personal learning from your placement.

Personal evaluation of the placement and of your learning is important regardless of whether you passed or failed the placement.

Table 18.1 Reflection on your placement

1	Did I prepare myself adequately for the placement? Did I check out the requirements, read up about the clients and conditions and develop my knowledge base adequately? In what way might these preparations have been more thorough?
2	Was my learning contract (or were my learning objectives) realistic? How might they have been different?
3	Did I take appropriate responsibility for achieving identified goals? Should I have done more, or done things differently?
4	Did anything interfere with my learning or achievement of my goals? Could I have managed any situation better?
5	Having identified my strengths, how will I build on these in the future?
6	What was the essence of the constructive advice given in the evaluation of this practice? How might I use this in the future?
7	What have I identified as my learning needs for my next placement?

Table 18.2 Personal learning from your placement

1	What have I learnt from this fieldwork experience: about the client group? about the service, its organization and delivery? about working in this particular field? about working with the team? about myself?
2	Have I gained in confidence and how?
3	Have I surprised myself with anything I have done and in what way?
4	In what way am I more competent in my skills and practice? What brought this about?
5	Which of my personal skills and qualities need further development?
6	What are my next learning goals?

Follow this through by writing down your responses to the questions in these two tables and then discuss them with colleagues in a debriefing session, or informally with a friend in your own time.

Evaluation helps develop an understanding of the consequences of decisions and actions. It helps to identify what works well, what does not work well in practice, and in what circumstances. This is how clinical reasoning develops. Paying attention to the evaluation of practice helps with the progression from a novice towards an expert practitioner.

It is important for students to become self-disciplined in preparation for professional life and to develop effective means of judging information and knowing how to use it discriminately in practice. Improved professional practice, client care and service delivery can result from systematic evaluation of performance. As we have noted in earlier chapters, developing sound evaluation skills allows you to contribute effectively to your own personal appraisal, to peer review and to service audit.

DEBRIEFING

Meeting up with your student colleagues again after your fieldwork experience can be very exciting. There will be plenty of news to exchange and experiences to share. You are all likely to have been changed both personally and professionally by the fieldwork experience and this needs to be acknowledged. You may recognize changes in your colleagues and how they present in confidence, maturity and their understanding of practice. Your colleagues may identify similar changes in you. You will learn a good deal from informal discussions with your peers but certain issues need to be explored more formally in debriefing sessions.

Discussions need to be guided to ensure constructive use is made of all your observations about the fieldwork experience. Returning to the academic setting can seem pretty mundane after the excitement of practice, but it is important to set the fieldwork experience into context and relate the learning which has taken place to the total educational programme. Links need to be made between theoretical knowledge and practice, between simulated and real-life environments and between the ideal or potential of service provision and the reality in practice.

For the debriefing, you will probably convene in small discussion groups to hear about others' experiences, challenges and learning, as well as to talk about your own fieldwork practice. You will hear about the variety of Occupational Therapy services and the demands made of practitioners in the different settings. You will be alerted to the varying quality of fieldwork educators, fieldwork supervision and fieldwork education. A good facilitator will ensure that the discussions remain constructive and that principles learned from the various experiences are drawn to your attention.

Some students will have had good experiences, others not so good. This may be the time to reflect on the amount of personal responsibility that students are expected to take for ensuring a positive fieldwork placement. Remember as you listen to your colleagues in the debriefing sessions that only the student's perspective is represented. There are often two sides to a story. As fieldwork educators are not present to put forward their views you may need to reserve your judgement of a given situation. You would be better advised just to examine the principles and processes of the experience, for future reference.

SUPPORTING COLLEAGUES WHO HAVE FAILED

Some of your colleagues may need support if they have failed on a placement or have had a particularly bad experience. They may need reassurance about their potential to become an occupational therapist. Failing a placement can be a personal blow, prompting a good deal of self-searching and examination of contributory factors. After a placement some students realize that Occupational Therapy is not, after all, the career for them and they choose to leave the course. For others, it takes longer to understand and adjust to the demands that the profession is making of them. A second chance to undertake the placement can be valuable in providing that extra time to adjust and come to terms with what is required.

SUMMARY

The evaluation of learning should not be left to chance. A structured approach to evaluating the learning experience is an essential component of that experience.

Informal discussions and sharing the experience with colleagues are valuable for learning. Formal debriefing in the university will set that learning into the context of the total professional education programme. Principles of learning and plans for future action can then be formulated.

19 Researching practice

This chapter covers:

- the purpose and historical development of research in professional practice;
- levels of research;
- case studies and case stories;
- ethical considerations.

> We will achieve recognition as a true profession and academic discipline only if we are committed individually and collectively to the importance of scientific inquiry and scholarly activity (p. 215).

These challenging words by Ottenbacher (1987) urge occupational therapists to be proactive and forward thinking about conducting research in order to build on their successes and correct their failures. These days it is vital that we substantiate what we are doing in practice through research. Citing 'custom and practice' is no longer sufficient. Increasingly, quality control and cost containment are influencing the way we work (Ong, 1993). As a result, purchasers of health services, may only choose to buy services which have been found, through research, to be effective. Some elements of our practice which we have always believed to be sound, but have never proved to be effective may ultimately be rejected.

An example which illustrates this point comes from the USA. The Federal Agency for Health Care Policy and Research (AHCPR, 1995) recently issued a set of guidelines for post-stroke rehabilitation. Because of lack of research, neurophysiologically and neurodevelopmentally based treatments for restoration of motor control were not included. This makes quite a statement about an area of practice in which many therapists work. It has prompted the profession to take action (Trombly, 1995).

On placement you may well be required to carry out some project work as part of your course, or at your fieldwork educator's request. The work may involve presenting a case study or a case story drawn from fieldwork, or a larger research project which forms part of your academic course work. In this chapter we focus on the kinds of studies which you might have to undertake during your fieldwork education, but before we go into detail, we would like to look first at what research is, and then at the historical development of research within the profession.

WHAT IS RESEARCH?

According to Bailey (1991) research is any activity undertaken to increase our knowledge; it is the systematic investigation of a problem, issue or question. Payton (1994) defines it as the goal-directed process of looking for a specific answer to a specific research question in an organized, objective and reliable way. It is not just a search for what others have already discovered but a rigorous search for new knowledge. Payton suggests that research is the discovery and validation of the concepts and principles on which our practice is based and argues that future health professionals must be prepared to defend, with rational and scientific evidence, the appropriateness (i.e. the validity) of their practice and procedures. These comments suggest that research is an essential professional activity and if we wish to continue to call ourselves 'professionals' we must take steps to expand the profession's body of knowledge which underpins its practice. We must use research to provide the evidence that occupational therapists' work is beneficial to clients and that our practice is efficient and effective.

Hopkins and Smith (1993) propose that research is important for three main reasons.

1. It develops and extends the knowledge base of the profession.
2. It contributes to the development and validation of Occupational Therapy tests and measurements (and, we would argue, other areas of practice).
3. It documents the effectiveness of Occupational Therapy interventions.

The important point is the documentation of the results. Communication of results is an often neglected stage of the research process but it is essential to publish findings and make them available to others so that the work can be drawn upon to inform future practice and subsequent research studies. The Code of Ethics and Professional Conduct for Occupational Therapists (College of Occupational Therapists, 1995) places a responsibility on members of the profession to contribute to the continuing development of the profession by critical evaluation, audit and research, and to base practice on established research findings. Research must therefore been seen as integral to practice. In the next section we examine the historical development of research within the profession.

Historical development of research

Research is linked to academic progress, and currently there is an upward trend in professional education from diploma to first degree, and to continuing postgraduate studies at master's and doctoral level, and beyond. Master's degrees in Occupational Therapy began in the 1960s in the USA and this is why many major research studies, the majority of models of practice and most textbooks have come from there in the past. We can now expect a change in this trend as occupational therapists from other countries gain higher degrees and produce published work.

Most early studies in the 1960s and 1970s were conducted during the period when Occupational Therapy was firmly entrenched in the medical model of practice. Therapists worked predominently in hospitals, so many studies at this time were medically and scientifically orientated. Research methods followed scientific methods which were quite precise and studies tended to focus on defined areas of work, often related to specific parts of the body. Somehow this scientific method of research did not fit with the holistic vision of the occupational therapist and it may account for the dearth of research in mental health practice.

Increasingly scholars became uncomfortable with scientific methods. Neistadt (1988) for instance, questioned the way in which perceptual deficits in people who had suffered a cerebral vascular accident (CVA) were being examined. At about the same time, Nedra Gillette, who headed the American Occupational Therapy Foundation (AOTF) for research development, suggested that other research methods might be more appropriate for occupational therapists. In the late 1980s the first studies to examine the clinical reasoning of occupational therapists were taking place. These studies were conducted by an anthropologist who used action research and ethnographic methodology for her work (Mattingly and Gillette, 1991). Qualitative methods used routinely in the social sciences suddenly became legitimate in Occupational Therapy research. It was realized that this approach seemed to be much more appropriate for many of the studies that the profession wanted to conduct.

A marked change in the studies that have been published over the past few years can be seen from reading the *American Journal of Occupational Therapy*. Fleming (1991) compared the differences between research in medicine to that in Occupational Therapy. Therapists were becoming known either as **quantitive** scientific researchers or **qualitative** naturalistic researchers, which prompted Gillette (1991) and Ottenbacher (1992) to write about this trend. Ottenbacher and Petersen (1985) had already examined the differences between articles written in the *American Journal* between 1973 and 1983. They noted that articles were increasingly written by therapists with higher degrees, that the studies were more sophisticated in design and that they were often written by multiple authors, showing a trend towards collaborative research.

Articles also progressed from those where no statistics were used, to descriptive statistics, and from elementary statistics to advanced statistics. Ottenbacher and Petersen also pointed out that not only was it essential for therapists to do research, it was also necessary for them to be able to understand published papers otherwise research findings could not be incorporated into their practice. This historical account demonstrates the need for research, and for a base of knowledge to validate Occupational Therapy practice.

Choice of method

Choice of research method ultimately depends on **what** you choose to research and not on whether you favour qualitative or quantitative methods. For this reason you need to be aware of someone who espouses one method to the exclusion of others, and feels that theirs is the method of choice. You should examine critically what is to be researched and define the methodology which best suits that study. You should also be aware that one criticism often levelled at qualitative research, compared with the scientific method, is its lack of rigour. If you are contemplating research using any of the qualitative methods we would recommend that you read

Krefting's (1991) paper which details the criteria for trustworthiness of this form of enquiry.

Research methods are now part of every undergraduate course. There are many books and papers on research methods so we do not go into detail here. We do suggest, however, that you look at the date of publication of the book or article that you are consulting. Check the background of the author(s) to see if they come from the therapy professions, social sciences or other fields and look at the qualifications of the writer(s) to determine their experience and the research studies which they have carried out. This may help you to select the literature that will serve you best.

LEVELS OF RESEARCH

The term 'research' can seem quite frightening especially when you find out that you have to carry out a study as part of your undergraduate course. But at this level you are merely practising using the research process and learning what it is like to be a researcher, you are not expected to take on a major life-long task! Barnes (1995) offers students sensible advice about choosing and carrying out research at this level, but the key to success of a project is to keep it small and simple.

As you progress through your course and go beyond it, your level of professional knowledge will grow. You will acquire additional skills and experience, and your ideas will develop. Many of you, hopefully, will go on to enrol for Master's programmes and a small proportion of you will contemplate PhD studies. You might not wish to think that far ahead at the moment, as you grapple with the complexities and demands of your undergraduate course, but the opportunities are there and you should not be afraid of taking them. Any project that you carry out at undergraduate level will therefore provide practice for later research.

The profession needs researchers at all levels and just as your professional knowledge and skills will grow, so will your ability to do research. There are several levels of research each with different expectations but as Bell (1993) points out, the issues to be addressed are much the same whether you are producing a small scale project, a Master's dissertation or a PhD thesis. Each involves:

- selecting a topic of interest;
- identifying the objectives;
- designing a suitable methodology (giving consideration to ethical issues);
- devising the research instrument(s);
- negotiating access to resources;
- collecting, analysing and presenting data;
- producing a well-written report.

In the next few paragraphs we outline very briefly the usual expectations at different levels of research so that you can gain an appreciation of where the undergraduate project stands in the research continuum. We then provide some guidance on how you might approach case studies and case stories which often have to be completed during fieldwork education and which are more likely to feature in undergraduate programmes.

The undergraduate project

Projects are normally associated with courses at diploma or first degree level. Analytical rigour is not usually demanded, although some evidence of ability to analyse will certainly be expected of occupational therapy students. Independent enquiry and exercise of judgement is, however, required, as is a reasonable standard of presentation of results. At this level, students can expect to complete a project report. This will be a well structured and convincing account of the study showing the resolution of the problem addressed (Howard and Sharp, 1983) with adequate reference to literature.

Postgraduate dissertations

Studies for post-graduate diplomas or taught master's degrees will include an element of independent research which is reported and presented as a **dissertation**. At this level the student would be expected to use research methods, handle data and recognize shortfalls in the research process. The dissertation will be an ordered, critical and reasoned exposition of knowledge which shows evidence of good use of literature (Howard and Sharp, 1983).

Master's degrees by research

According to Phillips and Pugh (1994) the award of a Master's degree marks the possession of advanced knowledge in a specialist field. In historical terms a master's degree was always considered a licence to practise (originally to practise theology). A master's degree by research is awarded on the basis of a **thesis** which is a coherent extended account of a significant research project which shows some originality. The term thesis comes from the Greek language and means argument (Barnes, 1995) which gives you an idea as to what might be expected. The researcher must show competence in the independent execution of the work, an understanding of appropriate techniques and the ability to make critical use of published work. Some appreciation of the relation of the special theme to the wider field of knowledge is normally required (Howard and Sharp, 1983). Conducting a study at this level is often deemed to be the apprenticeship for PhD studies.

Doctoral studies

Where a master's degree has historically been held to be a licence to practice, a doctor's degree is considered a licence to teach. As an anomoly, medical practitioners hold honorary doctorates through which they have achieved licence to practise. Someone with a doctorate is recognized as an authority by the relevant faculty, and as someone who has attained the status of a professional researcher. Those who study at this level are expected, through their research, to make a significant and original contribution to their chosen field and to add to the body of knowledge in a way that has not been done before (Phillips and Pugh, 1994). The examination is by thesis and by an oral defence of that thesis.

The above are broad descriptions of studies at the different levels. Each university and each course will have its own criteria for the conduct and presentation of research at the different levels and these should be your main guide. We make no apology, however, for presenting the different levels. Just as we explained the journey from novice to expert practitioner in Chapter 14, here we show you the progression from novice to professional researcher so that you can see how it fits with your ideas about professional development. As a final comment in the review of levels, Table 19.1 shows the expectations of students in the caring professions at different levels. The material has been drawn from discussions with representatives of social work, Occupational Therapy and nursing professions.

CASE STUDIES AND CASE STORIES

Research is often thought of as a scientific process which requires a strict, rigorous approach and which results in a flawless piece of work. While scientific methodology does require some precision, not all research has these characteristics. Some research which aligns with the qualitative approach is less structured, but even so must be trustworthy. Examples are case studies and case stories which you might be asked to complete as part of your course requirements. Denzin (1989) makes a distinction between the two. Case studies comprise the sequence of events using official material which is truthful, accurate and verifiable, and which omits the subject's account. Case stories embrace the subject's interpretations of, and reactions to events which have taken place. The meaning of events for the subject is important as it sheds light on the actual experience. The next sections explain the characteristics of case studies and case stories in more detail.

Case studies

There are different interpretations of the term case study.

1. In its simplest form, a case study may involve investigating and presenting the case of a client with whom you have been working and in whom you have taken a special interest. The case study may be written as a report or presented orally to a group of people. Occupational Therapy programmes often have their own guidelines for preparing the case study material. For a case study you will normally be expected to explore the client's situation by reading his/her records and notes, analysing and reflecting on the reports of the client's progress, talking to the client and his or her carer and to the personnel who have been involved in the client's care management. It will be important to search out relevant background information, to discover the client's and carer's views, perspectives and expectations for the future, and to present a critical account of the care management process. An evaluation of intervention and how effective it was will probably be expected. A general format for presenting case studies is given here. It will probably contain the following points

(a) details of client's history: age, sex, marital status, medical diagnosis, current treatment setting, recent precipitants for admission or referral, previous living situation, life roles, interests, accomplishments and functional status and family and social supports;

Table 19.1 Expectations of students: research levels

The developing professional should:			
At Foundation level	At Diploma/BSc level	At MSc level	At M.Phil/PhD level
1. Know how to study	1. Know how research underpins professional thinking and practice	1. Have a repertoire of research skills	1. Be able to carry out original work independently
2. Know how to search in a library	2. Be able to use selected/descriptive research methods	2. Be able to draw on various research designs	2. Make critical use of published work (primary sources)
3. Know how to handle data	3. Be able to critique, compare and contrast pieces of work	3. Show competence in the use of selected research methodology	3. Be able to develop sophisticated theoretical arguments
4. Know about ethical issues	4. Be able to use literature to underpin arguments and analysis	4. Show evidence of wide reading	4. Provide new insights; develop new theory
5. Know how to plan a research project	5. Be able to present balanced arguments	5. Be able to integrate theory into analysis and evaluation	5. Demonstrate mastery of research processes and techniques
	6. Be aware of alternative perspectives	6. Be able to advocate new solutions to current problems	6. Make a significant and original contribution to the chosen field
	7. Be able to reflect on his/her work and integrate personal observations into written work	7. Be able to develop theoretical knowledge	7. Be able to defend orally the research undertaken
		8. Present abstract personal constructs and theories	
		9. Be able to develop and use different perspectives	
		10. Be able to critically evaluate own work	

(b) client's goals, beliefs and concerns regarding the problems experienced, and the intervention;
c) Occupational Therapy goals and plan; the selected model or approach to treatment;
(d) motivational obstacles and client's response to intervention;
(e) evaluation of the case and the management of the client's care.

Students are often asked during fieldwork to present a case study as described above. There are, however, other types of case study which you might be required to undertake. Two are described briefly below.

2. According to Payton (1994) nominal descriptive research, often called a case study, is an approach that you might take when you know almost nothing about a defined topic of interest. One or several pre-planned observations of the 'case' are made. They are pre-planned because you will already have defined what you are looking for, how you are going to look for it, and how you are going to record your observations. You might study a client's case in detail because the case was interesting or unusual and for this you would:

- observe the client carefully on a number of occasions;
- make detailed notes of the client's behaviour, typical as well as atypical;
- note what prompts particular behaviours;
- refine the study to include measurements of specific elements if necessary.

Using this method you would then write a detailed account of your observations from which you would identify, describe and evaluate the essential characteristics of the case and behaviour under scrutiny.

3. Yin (1984) advocates that the case study method can be used to study a single case or small number of cases in depth within a particular context in order to capture 'still frames' of an organization at a moment in time. The method might be one to choose where the meaning and significance of the issue that you are studying are determined largely by the situation (Jankowicz 1991). Jankowicz sees an advantage of the case study over other methods, as in the case study the researcher describes and analyses the full richness and variety of events and issues occurring in the organization in question. It is by studying a single case in depth that provides greater understanding and insights into a defined situation. Results of case studies are, however, not readily transferable to other 'cases' as each will be bound by context. Insights gained from the study do, however, add to a knowledge base.

Case stories

A case story is a way of discovering and presenting information about a client and determining a course of action based on a perceived future life story. A case story might contain the following points.

1. An image of the client; a record which tells the client's story including details of:

- events which led to the client's contact with a health professional;
- the client's experience of the episode in his/her life and the meaning that it held for him or her;

- the cultural, social, spiritual and environmental context of, and influences on, the client's situation.

2. A critical appraisal of the options for intervention, taking into account the client's prospective, or future, story. This will revolve around history and prognosis. It will also relate to the picture formed of the client's future, and his/her potential for managing changes in his/her life.
3. A critical account of the intervention which shows how the client's perspective was used to inform the therapeutic programme.

These are just a few of the possible types of studies which you might choose or be required to carry out in the fieldwork setting. But whatever the study there are likely to be ethical issues to consider.

ETHICAL CONSIDERATIONS

Ethical principles

The question of ethics is essentially about what is right and what is wrong for researchers to do in pursuit of their goals (Haworth, 1993). Over recent years a number of articles have been written which address the issue of ethics in practice (Barnitt, 1993a, 1993b, 1994; Neuhaus, 1988). Discussions about ethical principles are now on the agenda of most Occupational Therapy programmes. Ethics in relation to research is governed by guiding principles similar to those in practice, for instance:

1. The Principle of Beneficence:

- freedom from harm;
- freedom from exploitation;
- benefits from research;
- the risk/benefit ratio.

2. The Principle of Respect for Human Dignity:

- the right to self-determination;
- the right to full disclosure;
- issues relating to the principles of respect.

3 The Principle of Justice:

- the right to fair treatment;
- the right to privacy.

Davis (1986) summarizes the basic ethical principles as: do no harm, be faithful to contracts and do all one can for the patient. As Payton (1994) suggests, there are three questions for the researcher to ask:

1. Am I trying to do good to the patients?
2. Am I respecting the freedom of choice that each patient has by right?
3. Am I being fair to everyone concerned with this project?

The first question challenges the researcher not merely to justify that no harm is being done but to identify that some good will actually come from the project. You should remember that the clients you work with in the fieldwork situation are in a vulnerable position because of what has happened to them and in all circumstances, morally and legally, you owe them a duty of care. You must therefore make every effort to respect their rights and privacy. Clark (1993) and Whitney (1995) describe research from the client's perspective and note how therapists should behave. Before you embark on any research project you must therefore consider the ethics of your project and the effect that it might have on those involved. Gathering information for simple case studies or case stories may not need approval of an ethics committee but the consent of the client concerned should always be sought.

Ethics (human subject) committees

Ethics committees are established by organizations to vet and approve research study proposals. Through this process they protect the interests of clients, patients and staff who might be asked to engage in the research process. Committees within health services in the UK are generally known as ethics committees. Other countries such as the USA use the term 'human subjects committee'. In England and Wales there is also the Services Evaluation, Research and Information Committee which vets all research proposals on behalf of local authorities (Association of Directors of Social Services, 1992). We note the address of this committee in Appendix A.

Ethics committees, as part of their remit, assure themselves that researchers will take steps to inform subjects fully of the nature of the research project in which they have been invited to take part. Individuals can then make an informed decision about whether to agree or decline to participate in the study. Subjects who agree to take part thus give **informed consent**.

Informed consent

Bailey (1991) defines informed consent as consent freely given by a participant in a research project based upon full disclosure of the procedures that the individual will undergo (p. 205). The consent form or letter should be written in terms which are comprehensible to the layman and should include all the information about the study that any reasonable person would need or want to know. The form or letter should avoid persuasion and should not raise false hopes. Every effort should be made to ensure that participants fully understand what is intended in the research. They should not be feel coerced in any way into taking part (Haworth, 1993). Sometimes a judgement has to be made about whether a person is able to understand sufficiently to be able to give consent, for instance a person with learning difficulties or mental health problems. It may be desirable or necessary to approach someone who can act on the client's behalf to consider the issue of consent. The emotional state of those who have agreed to take part also needs to be monitored and any subject showing signs of distress or discomfort in the course of the study should be withdrawn (Haworth, 1993). Your university may have a pro-forma from which you can compile a letter of consent which relates to your particular study. Other examples are to be found in Bailey (1991). It is sometimes considered better for a third party to approach the client with the letter so that he or she may feel free to refuse to take part in the study without fear of upsetting the researcher.

Ethical screening

Ethics committees in hospitals and those acting for local authorities are in place to protect the interests of staff and clients within their organization. As a student wishing to undertake research in one of these organizations, you may be required to submit a proposal to the appropriate committee, if your study involves human subjects. The academic staff at your university will advise you. Be warned, however, that ethics committees may only sit every two or three months so you will need to give yourself plenty of time to complete the vetting procedures before you start the project. If your study involves more than one agency, then both may need to be approached for permission. You may additionally, or alternatively, have to submit your proposal to a screening committee within the university. This may be a local arrangement for vetting students' research proposals instead of having them submitted to the health or local authority committee for approval. Pinnington and Bagshaw (1992) and Bagshaw and Pinnington (1992) describe the process of establishing an ethical screening procedure for a School of Occupational Therapy.

Taking photographs and videofilms

The fieldwork setting offers opportunities to photograph and video practice but before any such activity takes place it is essential to gain permission from every person who might appear on the film. Written consent is essential and the consent form will detail the exclusive purpose(s) for which the film or photograph would subsequently be used.

RESEARCHABLE TOPICS

If you have developed an enquiring mind you are unlikely to be at a loss for a topic to research. Researchable questions can come from many sources and areas of practice. The most important factors to consider are your own particular interest in the topic, the timescale in which you have to complete the project and the availability of, and access that you have to the resources that you need to complete it. You should look to your academic tutors to help you to define the research project so that it is relevant to your studies and manageable in the timescale.

The other thing to keep in mind is that the research project is **your** project. You will own it. For this reason you should be guarded about anyone in the fieldwork situation wishing to influence your choice of study. Other people may have their own reasons for wanting a particular project carried out and may want to use the material subsequently for their own purposes. Some practitioners, who are less experienced in research may try to guide you into undertaking a project which is too large for the purpose of your degree studies. By all means listen to what is being suggested, but do take responsibility for your work and ensure that you are able to meet the criteria for your degree.

Developing your research ideas

It is not within the scope of this book to examine different research methodologies. You should seek advice from your research supervisor about your particular study especially if you are embarking on research for the first time. Once you have decided on your topic you can take steps to gain further information. This may include making an on-line library search for literature to enhance your knowledge base and accessing research networks and data bases across the country, including those of the professional organization. A good deal of research is never published. It is left in thesis form and only registered in local library data-bases so these are also worth checking. We have included Table 19.2 to guide you as you work on your project. Go through the criteria systematically as you plan your project, and again after you have written it up to see if you have met each criterion.

Contact with researchers

During your training you may come into contact with a variety of people who are carrying out research. Your lecturers may be undertaking studies, either for higher awards or as part of their professional work. Your fieldwork educators, other occupational therapists, members of other professions or service managers may be undertaking, or be somehow involved in, research studies. Use any opportunity that you can to find out what these people are doing, why they settled on a particular topic, how they refined their research questions, what methodology they chose to use, what problems they encountered and how they resolved them. Most people enjoy talking about their projects. Their enthusiasm and motivation can be infectious and inspire those around them to engage in the research process. Do see these as learning opportunities. Note their observations about the research process because these may be pertinent when you come to undertake your own study.

Increasingly these days Occupational Therapy departments accepting students for placement have research high on their agenda. Occupational therapists as part of everyday practice are engaged in research as an expectation of their service employer. This means that exposure to research by every Occupational Therapy student who works in that setting becomes the norm. Students have the opportunity to observe and/or participate in a research study, and research issues are covered as an integral part of the fieldwork programme. An example of such practice is described by Mauras-Neslen and Robertson (1995). Centres in the UK can be expected to increase their research activity over the next few years as more funds become available for research projects. As a student you should ask what research activity is taking place so that you can gain experience and develop your research as well as your clinical skills.

Table 19.2 A guide to the development of your research project

Points to consider

Project Title: Student's Name:________________

Please rate each criterion:	Has met criterion		
	Yes	Needs revision	No
1. Understanding of scope of problem			
2. Delineation of a researchable question on topic			
3. Logical development of topic in each stage			
4. Appropriateness of methodology Comments:			
5. Accuracy of content			
6. Extent and depth of investigation			
7. Organization of content			
8. Clarity of presentation			
9. Evidence of original thinking			
10. Potential for integration into body of knowledge			

BENEFITS OF RESEARCH

Apart from the benefits to the profession there are many personal benefits to carrying out research. You will master the foundation skills that are necessary to carry out the project and you will develop your ability to analyse and interpret your findings. You will work with theories and gain background knowledge and understanding of the subject matter. You will also gain a sense of achievement in having completed your project. You will almost certainly grow in personal and professional confidence and you will become a more critical thinker and more self directed in your learning. You will develop stamina, the ability to reflect, and you will feel empowered in the knowledge that you are a member of the group of life-long learners. As Bailey (1991) says, research can be fun, exciting and fascinating. You may well start out by being appalled by the idea but you are likely to end up feeling proud of the results and having enjoyed the challenge. There is a great sense of satisfaction to be derived from completing an exacting, often complex, but always stimulating project. We hope that you will enjoy carrying out a study at undergraduate level and that it will lead to many more exciting research projects in the future.

SUMMARY

This chapter suggests that research is an essential element of professional practice in that it underpins and justifies the work undertaken by occupational therapists. Research can be undertaken at all levels of professional development although expectations are different for those studying for higher awards. Research at undergraduate level should be kept simple and small-scale, and aim to meet course requirements. In the fieldwork setting there are many opportunities for research. Some of the approaches that might be taken are discussed. Ethical issues are addressed. The chapter concludes by outlining some of the benefits to individuals who engage in the research process and it indicates the learning that might take place.

REFERENCES

AHCPR (1995) Publication No. 95-0662, US Government Printing Office, Silver Spring, MD.

Association of Directors of Social Services, 1992.

Bagshaw, A. and Pinnington, L. (1992) The outcome and implications of screening student projects for evidence of ethical reasoning. *British Journal of Occupational Therapy*, **55**(12), 453–6.

Bailey, D. M. (1991) *Research for the Health Professional, a Practical Guide*, F.A. Davis Company, Philadelphia.

Barnes, R. (1995) *Successful Study for Degrees*, 2nd edn. Routledge, London.

Barnitt, R. (1993a) What gives you sleepless nights? Ethical practice in occupational therapy. *British Journal of Occupational Therapy*, **56**(6), 207–12.

Barnitt, R. (1993b) Deeply troubling questions: the teaching of ethics in undergraduate courses. *British Journal of Occupational Therapy*, **56**(11), 401–6.

Barnitt, R. (1994) Truth telling in occupational therapy and physiotherapy. *British Journal of Occupational Therapy*, **57**(9), 334–40.

Bell, J. (1993) *Doing your Research Project*, 2nd edn. Open University Press, Buckingham.

Clark, F. (1993) Occupation embedded in a real life: interweaving occupational science and occupational therapy. *American Journal of Occupational Therapy*, **47**(12), 1067–78.

College of Occupational Therapy (1995) *The Code of Ethics and Professional Conduct for Occupational Therapists*.

Davis, C. M. (1986) The influence of values on patient care. In Payton, E. D. (ed.) (1986) *Psychosocial Aspects of Clinical Practice*, Churchill-Livingstone, NY.

Denzin, N. (1989) *Interpretive Biography*. Qualitative Research Methods vol. 17, Sage Publications, Newbury Pary, CA.

Fleming, M. (1991) Clinical reasoning in medicine compared with clinical reasoning in occupational therapy. *American Journal of Occupational Therapy,* **45**(11), 988–96.

Gillette, N. (1991) The challenge of research in occupational therapy. *American Journal of Occupational Therapy,* **45**(7), 660–2.

Haworth, G. (1993) *Ethical Issues in Student Research in Occupational Therapy*. Christ Church College, Canterbury.

Hopkins, H. and Smith, H. (eds)(1993) *Willard and Spackman's Occupational Therapy*, 8th edn. J.B Lippincott Company, Philadelphia.

Howard, K. and Sharp, J. A. (1983) *The Management of a Student Research Project*. Gower, Aldershot, Hants.

Jankowicz, A. D. (1991) *Business Research Project for Students*, Chapman & Hall, London.

Krefting, L. (1991) Rigor in qualitative research: The assessment of trustworthiness. *American Journal of Occupational Therapy*, **45**(3), 214–22.

Mattingly, C. and Gillette, N. (1991) Anthropology, occupational therapy, and action research. *American Journal of Occupational Therapy*, **45**(11), 972–8.

Mauras-Neslen, E. and Robertson, S.C. (1995) Fieldwork NIH Style, *OT Week*, 18 May, 18–19.

Neistadt, M. (1988) Occupational therapy for patients with perceptual deficits. *American Journal of Occupational Therapy*, **42**(7), 434–41.

Neuhaus, B. (1988) Ethical considerations in clinical reasoning: the impact of technology and cost containment. American Journal of Occupational Therapy, **42**(5), 288–95.

Ong, B. N. (1993) *The Practice of Health Services Research*, Chapman & Hall, London.

Ottenbacher, K. and Petersen, P. (1985) Quantitative trends in occupational therapy research: Implications for practice and education. *American Journal of Occupational Therapy*, **39**(4), 240–6.

Ottenbacher, K. (1987) Research: its importance to clinical practice in occupational therapy. *American Journal of Occupational Therapy*, **41**(4), 213–15.

Ottenbacher, K. (1992) Confusion in occupational therapy research: does the end justify the method? *American Journal of Occupational Therapy*, **46**(10), 871–4.

Payton, O. (1994) *Research: The Validation of Clinical Practice*, 3rd edn. F.A. Davis Company, Philadelphia.

Phillips, E. M. and Pugh, D. S. (1994) *How to Get a PhD*, 2nd edn. Open University Press, Buckingham.

Pinnington, L. and Bagshaw, A. (1992) The requirement for ethical reasoning in occupational therapy education. *British Journal of Occupational Therapy*, **55**(11), 419–22.

Trombly, C. A. (ed.) (1995) *Occupational Therapy for Physical Dysfunction*, 4th edn. Williams & Wilkins, Baltimore.

Webster's Ninth New Collegiate Dictionary (1987) A Meriam-Webster Inc. Massachusetts.

Whitney, R. (1995) Don't say you know how I feel: a client's perspective. *OT Week,* 6 July, 20–1.

Yin, R. K. (1994) *Case Study Research: Design and Methods*, 2nd edn, Sage, Beverly Hills, Calif.

Becoming qualified

20

This chapter covers:

- managing the transition from Occupational Therapy student to qualified practitioner;
- choosing your first post;
- continuing your professional development

The Occupational Therapy curriculum and integral fieldwork components provide sufficient theoretical knowledge and experiential learning for you to become a competent practitioner. This book explains how the fieldwork elements play a significant part in that scheme of learning. It helps you explore how you might use these experiences to take control of your education and facilitate your own learning to qualifying level and beyond. Part of the responsibility of a professional is to continue that learning process after qualifying in order to maintain and improve skills and the ability to practise in a constantly changing environment.

Becoming an occupational therapist is both the end and the beginning of a stage in your career. It is a phase which involves transition (Bridges, 1980) where one life (as a student) gives way to another life (as a qualified practitioner) interceded by a temporary state of loss which Bridges calls the **neutral zone**.

Transition involves change. All through your studies an evolutionary process has been taking place. You have been exposed to many different experiences. You have drawn on your own experience of life prior to becoming a student to help you make sense of what has been happening in your studies. Gradually over the last few years you have taken on board many different aspects of the culture of your chosen profession and have prepared yourself for the new responsibilities of professional life.

Different people will notice changes in you and may well comment on how you seem to be different from when you embarked on your studies. Some may like the differences they perceive, others, particularly those closest to you, may be more reticent. You are no longer the person they once knew and this can affect relationships. Significant people in your life might actually prefer the person they once knew, others will be proud of what you have achieved and will support you as you take up your new role. Clearly you need to be sensitive to the way in which other people react to your qualification. Are you becoming more qualified than your partner for instance? Are you achieving greater earning capacity? How will your relationship be affected? These are matters you may need to address.

On your travels through your studies you will have learnt much about yourself. You will have come to recognize the strengths and limits of your own ability. You will have come into contact with a wide range of people from different cultures and backgrounds. You may well have had to question and perhaps adjust your values, beliefs, attitudes and understanding of people and situations. This exposure to the lives of clients as well as to organizational life will have left its mark. For you, any changes in the way you act and communicate may be imperceptible, for others, these changes may be blatently obvious. You need to consider carefully just how much you may have changed and what effect this may have on other people who are close by.

STUDENT TO EMPLOYEE

For qualifying occupational therapists, the change of status from student to employee has to be managed. Some have also to manage the change of status from Occupational Therapy assistant to occupational therapist and the change of working relationships that this entails. It can be an exciting time which often causes some anxiety, but it can also be a time of loss as student life is relinquished. The neutral zone, as Bridges (1980) puts it, is a temporary state of loss to be endured, a necessary kind of 'street-crossing procedure'.

After the rituals of end-of-course celebrations with colleagues and friends, there is a time when you might experience some emptiness in your life as the structure which supported your studies (and regulated your assessments!) disappears. It is understandable that this may be a relief for you, but it can also create loss of routine and associated loss in terms of friendship and support. This is the 'ending of an era' which requires some disengagement with the past. A new life is ahead of you which Bridges calls 'the new beginning' and which requires some kind of personal realignment in the face of uncertainty.

It is not unusual for finalist students to take 'time-out' at the end of their course to go on holiday or to take some significant break before moving into a new situation. This allows for some freeing up of time, for disassociating with the past, for revitalizing yourself and for allowing the transitional process to take its course.

YOUR FIRST POST

Many decisions have to be taken when it comes to searching for your first position as an occupational therapist. When should you start looking for a post? Where should you look? What should you look for?

When and where should you look?

It is quite common for students to start thinking about their first post at the beginning of the year in which they expect to qualify. The journals of Occupational Therapy will be full of adverts, job-shops may be arranged in your university and open days may be organized by individual services to tempt you to apply for vacant posts. In the foreseeable future there is likely to be a choice of posts, not only of first positions, but also of career opportunities within the profession. Posts become available throughout the year so there is no need to rush into making a decision. Take your time to identify exactly what it is that you want from the job (and what you do not want) before considering the options.

Some students make such an impact while undertaking fieldwork education within an Occupational Therapy service that they are encouraged to return to work for the service on qualification. This can be a real boost to confidence. Such a position may be attractive because you would be going back to a familiar situation to work with people who you know and have learned to respect – or would you? The Occupational Therapy workforce is very mobile with frequent staff changes. Restructuring of organizations is also a frequent occurrence so nothing remains the same. Do think very carefully about your needs and expectations if such a proposition is put to you. Consolidation of your practice in a familiar environment could be really rewarding but equally you should be aware of the potential for circumstances changing which might upset the balance of the situation. Some therapists actually choose to return to the site of their fieldwork experience to take up senior positions after gaining basic post-qualifying experience elsewhere. Think about this as an option before you commit yourself.

Where you seek your first position may be dictated by personal circumstances and where you choose to set up home. Many of you will be free to take up appointments anywhere in the country so you can consider many options. Others may be restricted by sponsorship contracts and a moral obligation to work for a sponsoring authority. The type of service and client group you wish to work with may also be factors in your decision about where to apply for jobs. Your choice of position may be influenced by your fieldwork experiences, by the type of clients you enjoyed working with on your placements, and by your particular strengths and abilities in dealing with the needs of these clients.

What should you look for?

Some of you might be quite clear about the field in which you want to work when qualified, others may be undecided. Some of you may be more clear about the field in which you do not want to work! Whatever the choice, there are some questions that you might consider asking at interviews to help you to decide.

1. *Will the position allow you to consolidate your learning in your chosen field? Are there opportunities for rotating into different areas of practice to gain further experience?*

   Opportunities for gaining rotational posts diminished with the creation of NHS Trusts. Services are more self-sufficient with fewer collaborative arrangements between Trusts. Opportunities for gaining experience in a range of areas have to be created in different ways which may be restrictive rather than facilitative of professional development.

2. *What opportunities are there for professional development?*

   Some larger organizations run in-service training schemes for newly qualified staff to facilitate their continuing professional development and preparation for career moves. Other organizations allow staff to apply in a rather ad hoc manner for courses which are likely to enhance service delivery to the client group served but not for courses which assist generally in personal and professional development. Some organizations offer very little in support of continuing staff development.

3. *How and with whom will professional supervision take place?*

   Increasingly Occupational Therapy services are managed by non-Occupational Therapy personnel and it may be important to you in your first post to ensure that you have access to profession-specific support, supervision and guidance.

4. *Is there a staff appraisal scheme in use?*

   During your professional education you will have learnt and applied skills of self-evaluation and reflection on your practice. These skills are important in all aspects of professional life. Appraisal schemes encourage you to use your reflective skills to review your professional performance, identify your professional development needs and agree an action plan for taking these forward. Professional supervision might help you in your day-to-day work but a more formal system of appraisal, sometimes known as Performance Review, can address wider development needs (Alsop, 1987). Where such schemes exist, you would be well advised to ascertain whether they are linked to salary reviews.

5. *What conditions of service apply?*

   Not only should you consider your salary, how it is reviewed and whether increments are awarded, you also need to consider other conditions of service. Where once many services were governed by nationally negotiated salary agreements, local pay bargaining is the current mode of decision-making about pay awards. You may be in a position to compare and contrast different conditions of service before accepting a post from those on offer to you.

   You might need to ask questions about annual leave, sick leave, maternity or paternity leave entitlement as these may vary. Conditions of service are increasingly governed by European law but they can still vary from service to service.

6. *Are you expected to use your car on duty for business purposes? Is a car lease scheme in existence?*

   Occupational therapists increasingly require transport to carry out their duties. Services tend to assume that you can drive and have a car which you are prepared to use for business purposes. Not everyone fulfils these criteria. Not everyone has a car which is not only road worthy but reliable. Not everyone would wish their car to be made available to people who are ill or dysfunctional. Not everyone keeps the inside of their car clean enough to be used for transporting relative strangers! Do check what is expected and consider whether you can accept the conditions imposed. Ask whether alternative schemes exist for booking, hiring or leasing transport to do the job.

7. *Will you be required to work 'unsocial' hours?*

   Opportunities to work 'unsocial hours' might be an advantage for you but you may need to check whether your managers are more likely to take advantage of you in asking you to work extraordinary hours! The norm is for Occupational Therapy to be available during normal 'office hours' although these may vary from place to place. Some services do offer 'out-of-hours' services – home visits and groupwork for instance. You need to gain clarity about what is involved, whether commitments are regular or arranged on a rota system, whether you are to get time off in lieu or additional payment for working these hours.

8. *Are there good working relationships between different professions or agencies?*

   Cooperation and communication between services and professionals is the foundation of good service delivery. You might like to ask not only whether this works but also for examples of how it works in practice. Collaboration and communication between professionals, however desirable, is never a foregone conclusion. You certainly would not want to take a first position and find yourself in conflict with others. Try to meet the team with whom you might work so that you can make up your own mind about the quality of work relationships that exist.

Remember when you are looking for a suitable position to use the interview situation to clarify points of concern. The interview is a two-way process and you should use it to assess the organization's potential for meeting your needs. You will find yourself drawing on many of your fieldwork experiences to inform the questions you ask. Once you have decided on a position and received your contract make sure that you understand and agree with everything in it and that any points of clarification or agreements reached at interview are reflected in the contract you receive.

WORKING INDEPENDENTLY

As you qualify and take responsibility as an autonomous health professional you will be practising without the degree of supervision that was available to you as a student. Clearly you need to ensure that you have some support in your new role, but the difference is that now you will be considered to be a competent practitioner who is able to work independently. It is worth keeping in touch with some of your student colleagues for continuing peer support to see you through the early weeks of employment. You might also keep in contact with your mentor.

CONTINUING PROFESSIONAL DEVELOPMENT

Your Occupational Therapy education will hopefully have inspired you to continue with your own professional development. Professional updating is a key responsibility of a practising health professional and one you should take very seriously particularly as it may become a requirement of continuing State Registration. Obviously there are many ways in which this can take place – through courses, workshops, in-service schemes, projects and so on. You should seriously consider keeping a portfolio as evidence of continuing professional development (Alsop 1995).

Those of you intent on a career within the profession should give serious consideration to developing a personal research profile. There is no need to start on a major research programme but do take an interest in research projects which others are carrying out and consider how you might develop some small project of your own. Your returning to higher education to teach, for instance, may depend on the strength of your research activity. The profession needs good researchers and pioneers who both challenge and confirm the boundaries of professional practice. Let us hope that you will be one of them.

FINALLY

Completing the Occupational Therapy programme and qualifying as an occupational therapist is a cause for celebration. After a period of consolidation of learning in your first post as an occupational therapist, we hope that you will then go on to develop your supervisory skills and become a fieldwork educator. You will be able to draw on your personal experience as a student, of fieldwork education and of your practice to fulfil a new, demanding but very necessary role. You will help to ensure the quality of fieldwork education for the next generation of students of the profession and enable them to qualify and join you in professional practice. We wish you luck in pursuing all your career aspirations and goals.

REFERENCES

Alsop, A. (1987) Why do we need staff performance review? *British Journal of Occupational Therapy*, **50**(3), 79–82.

Alsop, A. (1995) The professional portfolio: purpose, process and practice, part I: portfolios and professional practice. *British Journal of Occupational Therapy*, **58**(7), 299–302.

Bridges, W. (1980) *Transitions.* Addison Wesley, Reading, MA.

Appendix A

USEFUL ADDRESSES

Addresses of national professional associations

American Occupational Therapy Association, Inc.
4720 Montgomery Lane
PO Box 31220
Bethesda
Maryland 20824-1220
USA

British Association of Occupational Therapists/
College of Occupatonal Therapists
6–8 Marshalsea Road
Southwark
London SE1 1HL
UK

Canadian Association of Occupational Therapists
110 Eglinton Avenue
3rd Floor
Toronto
Ontario
Canada

Statutory body

Council for Professions Supplementary to Medicine
Park House
184 Kennington Park Road
London SE11 4BU
UK

Association of Directors of Social Services:
Service Evaluation, Research and Information Committee,
Assistant Director (Resources)
Hampshire County Council Social Services Department
The Castle
Winchester SO23 8UQ
UK

Appendix B

RELEVANT LEGISLATION IN THE UK

Professions Supplementary to Medicine Act 1960
Chronically Sick and Disabled Persons Act 1970
Health and Safety at Work Act 1974
Mental Health Act 1983
Data Protection Act 1984
Disabled Persons (Services Consultation and Representation) Act 1986
Consumer Protection Act (1987) Part 1 Product Liability
Access to Personal Files Act 1987
Education Reform Act 1988
Children Act 1989
Local Government and Housing Act (1989)
Access to Health Records Act 1990
National Health Service and Community Care Act 1990
Manual Handling Operations Regulations 1992

Index

Page numbers appearing in **bold** refer to figures and page numbers appearing in *italic* refer to tables.